Chiari M

Jennifer Wetzel, MA, May Chodron RN (Ed.),
Brian Hawking, MD (Ed.)

Copyright 2014 Jennifer Wetzel, MA, May Chodron RN, Brian Hawking, MD (Ed.). All rights reserved.

Cover photo: Valua Vitaly | Fotolia.com

ISBN 978-1497573482

Contents

Introduction 5
Anatomy of the Brain 17
Classification 29
Symptoms 33
Diagnostic tests 47
Treatment Options 55
How to find a Chiari surgeon 60
What Surgery is Like 62
Preoperative safety steps 71
Prognosis 77
Related Disorders 81
Ehlers-Danlos Syndrome 82
Fibromylagia 84
Hydrocephalus 86
Craniosynostosis 87
Endocrinopathy 87
Hyperostosis 88
Bone Mineral Deficiency 88
Cutaneous Disorders 88
Spinal Defects 89
Space-occupying Lesions 90
Glossary 93

Chiari Malformation Organizations 101

Internet Resources 103

Introduction

"I had a ridiculous, around-the clock migraine. I spent my days dizzy, in and out of blurriness and confused with a constant pressure in my head & neck. For years I took migraine pills, convinced I had the world's worst migraines. If only I had heard of Chiari malformation sooner, all those years of pain could have gone away..." Anne, Loveland CO.

Chiari malformation (CM), also called Arnold-Chiari, ACM I & II, hindbrain herniation or tonsillar ectopia, is a serious, structural condition that affects the base of the brain and skull. The area involved is where the spine joins the skull -- an area called the cranio-vertebral junction. The condition is named after Hans Chiari, an Austrian pathologist who reported the first incidence of Chiari malformation in 1891.

When the bottom part of the cerebellum -- the region of the brain that plays an important role in motor control -- expands out of the skull through the opening between the skull and the spine (the opening is technically called the foramen magnum), it forms what is called a *hernia*. A hernia is where an organ bulges out of the area it is supposed to be contained in. A hernia can happen to any organ, but when it affects the cerebellum it is called a Chiari malformation.

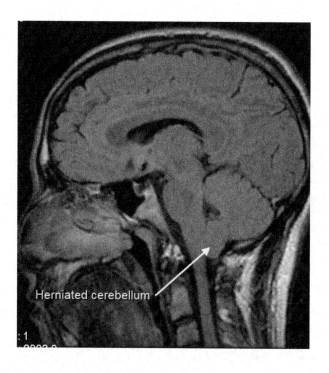

This bulge can cause serious issues, including many distressing symptoms such as severe headaches, balance problems, sleep disruptions, depression and incontinence. In addition, it can also cause a disruption in the flow of cerebrospinal fluid. This fluid normally acts as a cushion, protecting the brain and spine. Chiari malformation can also cause a compression in parts of the spinal cord.

The condition was once estimated to occur in one in a thousand births, although most of the cases are asymptomatic-- which means you technically have a CM but you don't have any symptoms like a headache or balance problems. However, due to the evolution of diagnostic imaging it is now thought to be a more common than originally thought. CMs are often detected by chance when a patient undergoes an MRI for an unrelated condition, such as head trauma after an accident. CMs are more common in women than in men, but it isn't understood why.

Exact figures of how many people are actually affected by this disorder are unknown. Complicating the estimation is the fact that many children who are born with CM will not show symptoms until their teenage years or early adulthood and many will never show symptoms at all. In other words, there could be many, many thousands of people with Chiari malformations who are blissfully unaware of their condition. This isn't necessarily a bad thing; even if you've been diagnosed with CM it doesn't necessarily mean you need treatment for it. In fact, for many people it never causes any problems, other than the psychological distress of knowing that there's something "wrong" with your brain.

"I was diagnosed with Chiari in 2001, after I was in a minor car accident and got whiplash. After I got the all-clear from an MRI (the whiplash just caused some muscle problems), I was horrified when my physician told me I had Chiari malformation. The thought that part of my brain was bulging out of my skull was so distressing at first that I felt I was in a constant state of panic – despite my doctor's reassurances that it might never cause any problems. Here I am more than a decade later, and I've never had a single symptom. The stress from the diagnosis went away after a few months, mostly after I did some research and found out it's a pretty common finding. I've almost forgotten about the diagnosis now!" – Julie, Miami FL.

If you have been diagnosed with Chiari malformation, or you have a relative who has been diagnosed, it's sometimes a very distressing diagnosis. There's something about having a problem with your brain that can make the bravest person quiver in their shoes. Add that to the fact that surgery is the only treatment for a symptomatic Chiari malformation (in other words, one that's causing symptoms), and you have what can seem like a daunting diagnosis. The thought of "brain surgery" is enough to induce stress in the calmest of people. There is good news; your CM may not need surgery if your symptoms are manageable. And if you *do* need surgery, you may not need actual surgery on your brain – you may be a candidate for surgery on just the skull itself (this procedure leaves the brain completely intact).

Why is surgery the only option for treatment?
You can think of it like a broken bone that's out of place; no medicine or homeopathic treatment will put the bone back where it's supposed to be. Surgery for many cases of CM consists of removal of a small piece of bone from your skull (a cranioectomy) to allow the cerebellum to return to a normal shape. The brain itself isn't actually touched for this procedure. For more invasive surgeries, surgery is on a very small portion at the base of your brain. In general, surgery has a good success rate – up to 80% of patients find their symptoms are relieved after surgery and severe complications are uncommon. For more information about the different types of surgery and possible complications, see the surgery section in the Treatments chapter later on in this book.

Causes

Chiari malformations can have many causes, including structural defects in the brain or spinal cord during fetal development in the womb. This type of CM is called primary or congenital CM and is the most common cause of CM. It is thought that congenital CM is caused by genetics (it's passed down through generations) or some cases may be due to inadequate maternal nutrition during pregnancy. In rare cases, high pressure inside the skull or very low pressure inside the spine can force the cerebellar tonsils downward. Another type of CM, called secondary or acquired CM can occur because the spinal fluid is drained excessively due to infection, exposure to toxins, or injury.

  The main reasons that researchers now think there is a genetic component to Chiari malformations include the fact that CMs are often seen in multiple family members. Plus, if one identical twin is diagnosed with CM Type I, then the other twin will also have the condition. CM Type I is known to co-occur with several different genetic disorders, which make researchers think there must be some kind of genetic connection.

  At the time of writing, the actual genes that may cause Chiari malformations have not been identified, and there is no available genetic test. However, there are some research studies underway to try and identify how CM is passed on through generations. For example, the Duke Molecular Physiology Institute is investigating this area for CM Type I with or without syringomyelia. Syringomyelia is a disorder commonly seen with CM where a fluid-filled cyst forms in the spinal cord. The institute is (as of April, 2014) recruiting families who have two or more family members with CM Type I. For more information, you can contact the institute at (919)-684-0655. A second study currently underway that is also investigating the genetic link for CM Type I is being conducted by the National Institutes of Health

Clinical Center in Bethseda, Maryland and at the Kazan State Medical University in the Russian Federation. If you have multiple family members affected and you are located either in the United States or in the Russian Federation, you may be a candidate for the research. You can contact the NIH Clinical Center at 800-411-1222 ext TTY8664111010.

Another clinical trial underway to attempt to better understand Chiari malformation is also being run by the NIH. The objective of the study is the conduct a 5-year natural history study of people with syringomyelia or a CM Type I (with or without syringomyelia). The study is an extensive one and includes:

- 7 outpatient visits to the National Institutes of Health Clinical Center: an initial visit; a visit 3 months later; and visits 1, 2, 3, 4, and 5 years after the initial visit. An additional 10 days of inpatient treatment and testing will be required if surgery is needed during the study.
- Medical history and physical examination.
- Detailed neurological history and examination.
- Blood and urine samples.
- MRI scans: Participants will have 2 scans at the initial evaluation, 2 scans at the 3-month visit, and 1 scan every year for the following 5 years.
- Additional neurological and imaging tests if needed, including a lumbar puncture to collect

spinal fluid, a myelogram (imaging study) of the spinal fluid, and a computed tomography scan of the skull and spine.

- Participants who are surgical candidates will have additional tests along with the surgery, including diagnostic studies (electrocardiogram and chest X-ray) before surgery and an MRI scan 1 week after surgery.

The contact for the natural history study is Gretchen C Scott, R.N. Her email is SNBrecruiting@nih.gov.

Research and studies are constantly being performed to find more information about Chiari malformation. Every year, something new is being discovered.

One fairly recent study (now closed to new patients) sought to find out if early surgical intervention in children makes a difference in outcomes. In other words, researchers wanted to know if earlier surgeries successfully resolved symptoms better than if surgeries were delayed until symptoms became more pronounced. The study was performed in children younger than 6 who had CM type I. The study identified 39 patients who had been diagnosed with this type of malformation before turning 6 and who had undergone surgery. After carefully analyzing their medical records, it was found that almost 80% of the children between the ages of 0 and 2 had a condition called oropharyngeal dysfunction, which is a difficulty with chewing and swallowing. Out of the children between the ages of 3 and 5, about 86% had syringomyelia, 38% showed scoliosis (a sideways bent spine), and 57% suffered from headaches. All the patients went through surgery, and in most cases, the surgery led to the resolution of the malformation or to a dramatic improvement of the initial symptoms. The study found that the early recognition of the disease together with the proper surgical treatment of Type I Chiari Malformation in children leads to good outcomes in most patients.

    Other studies have been performed in order to find out if early decompression of Chiari malformation in patients who also have syringomyelia resulted in stabilization or improvement of the associated scoliosis. The studies were based on the fact that CM Type I is often linked with scoliosis, particularly in infant patients. Past data showed that the incidence of scoliosis in patients with Chiari malformation and syringomyelia was higher in the infant population. About 82% of patients younger than 20 years with syringomyelia also had scoliosis, while only 16% of patients older than 20 years had the condition. Scoliosis in children can happen at very young ages and can progress very quickly. This particular study consisted of a twenty year review of surgical and nonsurgical treatment. All of the patients had gone through decompression surgery before turning 8. The research showed that scoliosis can improve dramatically after the decompression of CM Type I and that early decompression resulted in improvement or stabilization of the scoliosis. This eventually saved the patients from the need for spinal fusion, a surgical procedure that combines two or more vertebrae.

How to use this book

This book is intended as a guide for anyone who has been diagnosed with Chiari malformation, or for relatives of those diagnosed so that you can understand the condition. The first section of the book (anatomy) is a little dry, but necessarily so. We have tried to cut the medical jargon to a minimum so that you can see where the Chiari malformation is and why it produces so many symptoms.

The meat of the book is information about what symptoms you'll likely have, what you can expect during diagnostic procedures, and what surgery will entail. If you've never had surgery before, this can be a terrifying prospect (and so many people will put off surgery for years and years), so there is an expanded section on what you can expect from CM surgery to hopefully quash your fears and prepare you for making a decision about whether surgery is right for you. Some people are so terrified of surgery they would do anything to avoid it, and the suggestions in this book for non-surgical treatment may help you lift your quality of life to a level where you do not need surgery. In fact, it's possible in many cases of CM to permanently avoid surgery. Each person is different, but you may be one of the "lucky" ones who may never need to go under the knife.

"I had never had surgery before – not even dental surgery. The thought just made me sick to my stomach. I couldn't even think about surgery without having a panic attack. I think it was the thought of being out of control – asleep and maybe not waking up. I did eventually have surgery, and I honestly wish I had done it sooner. None of my fears about surgery turned out to be reality at all and my symptoms pretty much disappeared afterwards." Joe, Denver CO.

There are further sections on alternative and complementary medicine. However, it's important to note that these are only supplementary to the course of treatment that your physician recommends. A CM can't be "cured" with alternative or complementary medicine, but it can help you keep your symptoms under control.

We hope you find this book useful in your Chiari journey. At the very least, we hope that it will turn what can be a frightening diagnosis into one that you can make informed decisions about so that you can seek the right treatment for you and hopefully, conquer your Chiari.

Anatomy of the Brain

Although you can skip around this book and read it in no particular order, you might have a hard time truly understanding CM without a basic understanding of the parts of the brain that are affected. Feel free to skip this section if you don't want to read about anatomy right now – you can always refer back to it at a later time.

The Skull and Brain

Chiari Malformations involve an area at the back of the brain, where the skull meets the spine. The bone that covers the **cerebellum** (the part of the brain affected by CM) is called the **occipital bone**. When this bone (shaded in the next picture) is removed, it exposes the cerebellum.

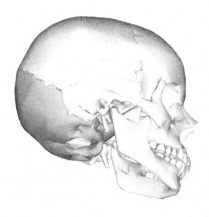

The following picture shows the occipital bone removed. In the center bottom is the **foramen magnum**, a hole which allows the spinal cord to pass through into the brain.

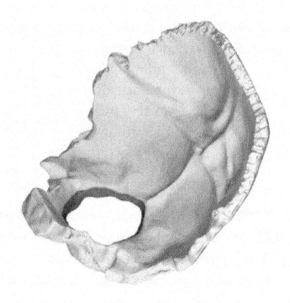

The part of the brain where the spinal cord connects is called the **brainstem**. It includes the midbrain, pons and medulla. The **midbrain** is a portion of the central nervous system associated with vision, hearing, motor control, sleep/wake, arousal (alertness), and temperature regulation. The **pons** is associated with sleep, respiration, swallowing, bladder control, hearing, equilibrium, taste, eye movement, facial expressions, facial sensation, and posture. The **medulla** contains the cardiac, respiratory, vomiting and vasomotor centers and is associated with breathing, heart rate and blood pressure.

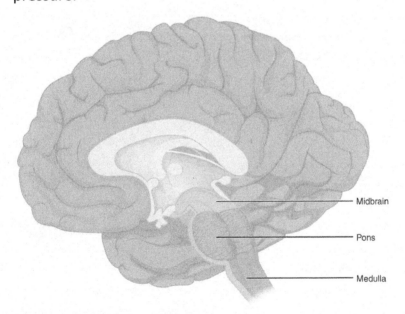

If you feel the back of your skull, there is a curved depression right above the spine. This area, called the **posterior fossa**, houses the cerebellum. In the following picture, you can see the posterior fossa at the base of the skull.

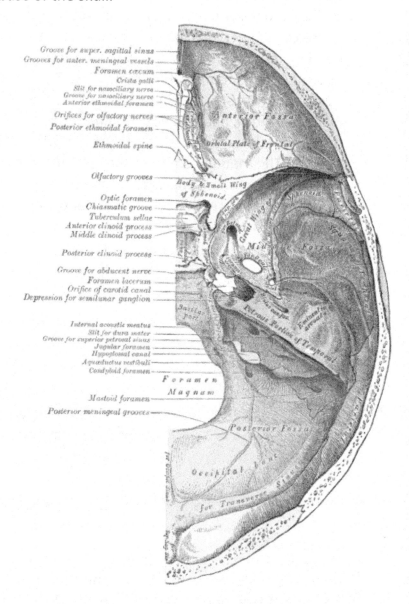

The **cerebellum vermis** is the middle part of the cerebellum. It regulates the muscles and influences attention, sensation, motivation, memory, behavior and autonomic activities like breathing, digestion and heart rate. The lateral (side) portion of the cerebellum is called the **cerebellar hemisphere**. This part is primarily involved in body movements, including fine motor movements.

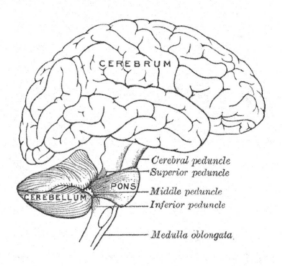

When the cerebellum passes through the foramen magnum, it's called a **cerebellar herniation**. The cerebellum can also be out of position (not protruding), a condition called **cerebellar ectopia**. You may have either one of these conditions with a Chiari malformation.

Another part of a Chiari malformation diagnosis involves the **cerebellar tonsils**. The cerebellar tonsils are located on the underside of the cerebellum. You can see the tonsils (not to be confused with the palatine tonsils at the back of your throat) at the center underside of the cerebellum in this next diagram, which is a cross-section of the cerebellum. The cerebellar tonsils are thought to influence limb movement and posture.

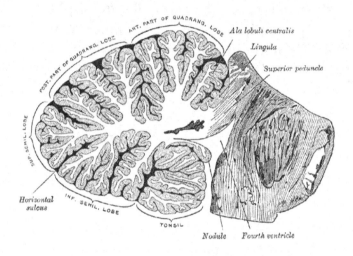

In a normal brain, the cerebellar tonsils are rounded. In a Chiari malformation, the tonsils can be squeezed out of the posterior fossa, into the spinal area and become pointed in shape.

When the cerebellar tonsils protrude through the posterior fossa, it's called a **tonsillar herniation.** When the tonsils are out of position (and not protruding), it's called **tonsillar ectopia**. Confusing the issue for Chiari malformation patients is this: even though the tonsils may be out of position, it may not produce symptoms (a condition called incidental or asymptomatic Chiari). Many people are thought to have this condition and never experience any symptoms. In other words, out-of-place tonsils or protruding tonsils may be considered a "normal" finding by your physician unless it is accompanied by Chiari symptoms. In addition, the size of the hernia doesn't equate to the severity of the symptoms. One patient with a small 3mm herniation may experience severe symptoms while another patient with a large 5mm herniation may experience no symptoms at all.

The Spine

The spinal areas involved in a Chiari malformation are the first two cervical vertebrae – the **atlas** and the **axis**. Those are the first two vertebrae at the top of your spine, where the spine meets your head. The atlas (shaded in the following picture) carries the weight of the head and is a ring-like structure. The axis is the next vertebrae down; it's the pivot on which the atlas rotates.

In some cases of CM, the atlas and the axis are fused together, preventing rotation of the head. In others, the **odontoid process** (the joint between the atlas and the axis) is not correctly aligned.

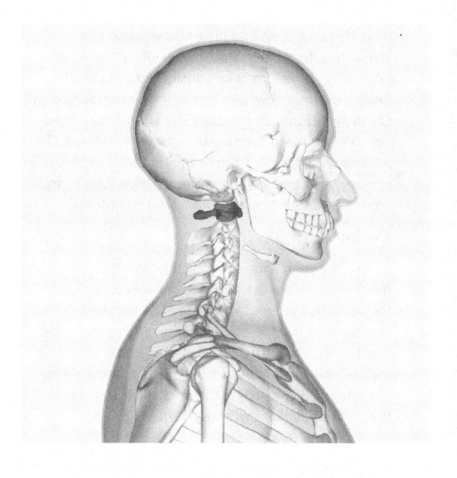

The spine (which includes the atlas and the axis) contains arteries and veins as well as the spinal cord, which carries the nerves. The spaces in the spine where the blood vessels are located are called **perivascular spaces**. These spaces are connected to the development of syringomyelia, a condition where a **syrinx** – a fluid filled sac – appears in the spine).

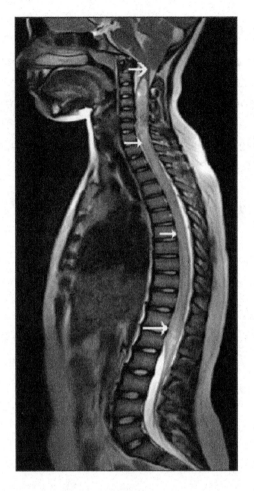

Image above: MRI showing Chiari I malformation (thick white arrow at the top) with a syrinx extending along the entire spinal cord from the axis to the conus medullaris (white arrow). The conus medullaris is the tapered, lower end of the spinal cord.

Cerebrospinal Fluid

Cerebrospinal fluid (CSF) is a clear fluid that bathes and protects the brain and spine. It gives a mechanical and immunological protection to the brain and provides a vital role in cerebral blood flow. The **meninges** (see next picture) are a protective layer for the brain and spine. CSF is located in the space between two layers of this protective layer called the **arachnoid** and the **pia mater**.

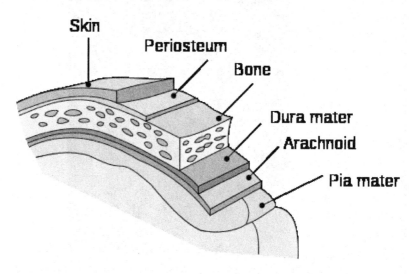

With Chiari malformation, the flow of cerebrospinal fluid can be disrupted or blocked. If you have a syrinx, the sac that forms in the spine is filled with cerebrospinal fluid.

The **fourth ventricle** is a cerebrospinal fluid filled space located behind the brainstem and just in front of the cerebellum. It's not to be confused with a syrinx, which is an abnormal fluid-filled cavity in the spine. The fourth ventricle is an essential component in the workings of the CSF system and is often involved in Chiari malformations. In the next image, the fourth ventricle is shown at the bottom:

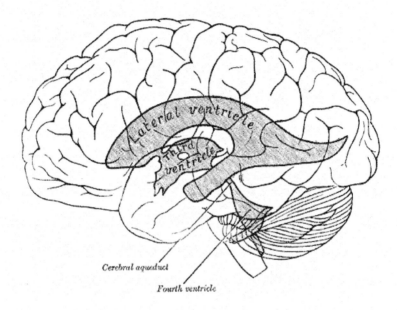

That's a basic overview of the brain and which parts of the brain, skull and spine that are involved in Chiari malformation. If you want to study these areas in more depth, we highly recommend Medline Plus (see Online Resources at the end of this book), an online government-run website that has hundreds of articles, videos and 3-D images of the human brain and associated conditions.

Classification

CMs are classified according to how severe the malformation is and which parts of the brain are protruding out of the skull. There are six main types:

Type 0

No protrusion is present, but the patient experiences CM symptoms, like severe headache. This type, which has a syrinx in the spinal cord, is currently under study and is a controversial diagnosis.

Type I

The lower part of the cerebellum protrudes into the foramen magnum. No symptoms may be present. This is the most common type of CM. A type I Chiari malformation is characterized by a downward displacement of the cerebellar tonsils of over 4mm. It's commonly diagnosed more in adults and teenagers than it is in children and is often found incidentally on an MRI due to investigation for another condition. Around 30% to 50% of patients with Type I have deformities of the skull and spine, which include:

- A bony union of the first vertebrae (the atlas) to the skull, or partial bony union of the first and second vertebrae.
- Scoliosis (curvature of the spine).
- Compression of the upper spine into the base of the skull.
- Cervical spina bifida occulta (a bony defect in the rear part of the spine).

Type II

The cerebellum and brain stem tissue protrude into the foramen magnum. This type is seen almost exclusively in patients with myelomeningocele, the most common type of spina bifida. It is a congential condition where the spinal cord and column do not close properly in the womb.

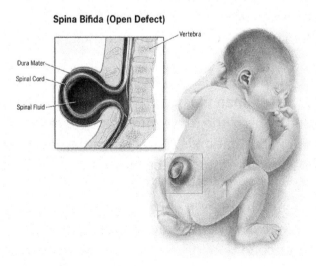

Additionally, the nerve tissue that connects the two halves of the cerebellum (the cerebellar vermis) may be absent or only partially complete.

Type III

The cerebellum and brain stem protrude into the foramen magnum. Part of the fourth ventricle – a fluid-filled cavity in the brain that circulates cerebrospinal fluid -- may also protrude. This is the most serious form of CM; it can cause severe neurological issues.

Type IV

A rare form of CM that involves an underdeveloped or incomplete cerebellum. This is the severest type and may accompany other malformations of the brain and brainstem. Most babies who are born with this type do not survive infancy. The cerebellar tonsils can be in a normal position and portions of the skull or spinal cord may be visible.

Women are affected by Chiari malformations more than men and certain groups are more susceptible. For example, people of Celtic descent are more likely to have a Type II malformation than members of the general population.

Symptoms

"I lived with my symptoms for nearly 30 years before getting a diagnosis. For the first 15 years, all I had were headaches (blinding, splitting headaches). Then, gradually I started to ache more in my limbs and experience pains in my legs. I thought they were related to growing older. In my mid-40s I began to experience chronic fatigue, sleeplessness, panic attacks and mild depression, which I chalked down to menopause. After I began to get tinnitus [ringing in the ears] and sleep apnea and after a ton of different diagnosis (including chronic fatigue) I was finally diagnosed with Chiari. What a relief! " Pam – London, Canada.

If you have Chiari malformation, it may cause a wide range of symptoms including:

- Depression
- Difficulty swallowing
- Dizziness
- Fatigue
- Headache in the back of the head which worsens when coughing or straining
- Hypersensitivity to bright lights
- Insomnia
- Mood changes
- Muscle Weakness
- Neck pain
- Loss of pain or temperature sensations in the upper body and arms
- Drop attacks (collapsing to the ground because of muscle weakness)
- Spasticity (an unusual tightness in your muscles)
- Blurred or double vision
- Numbness in legs or arms
- Problems with balance
- Problems with vision
- Respiratory (breathing) problems
- Ringing or buzzing in your ears or hearing loss
- Vomiting

"Over the years, I had definite symptoms that I brushed off because I thought – well, that's just life. I was "clumsy" – a sign that I wasn't balancing well...I also bumped into things a lot and dropped dishes or glasses on the floor. If something got broke in the house, I was always the culprit. But I thought I was just uncoordinated!" Dan, Middleburg FL.

Symptoms are different for every person and no set of symptoms can definitively say if you have Chiari or not. For example, even if you have the "classic" CM headache (a pressure headache at the back and sides of your head that can be excruciating), it doesn't mean that you have CM. It *could* be caused by low pressure in your skull, high pressure in your skull, a CSF leak (sometimes caused by epidurals during labor or neck trauma). It could also be caused by a plethora of other diseases and conditions, from the simple migraine to chronic conditions like fibromyalgia (see the "related conditions" chapter for more information). The possibilities are endless; only an MRI will reveal if you have a CM or not.

With type I, you may have no symptoms at all. If you do have symptoms, they normally appear no later than childhood or early adulthood. Sometimes, the symptoms may come on suddenly later in life, usually due to some kind of head or neck trauma. Although it's possible to have no symptoms at all, the vast majority of patients who do have symptoms report at least five of the above symptoms.

Type II and III are usually diagnosed at birth, or by an ultrasound during pregnancy. With Type II, you may have the above symptoms, but some symptoms are more common in type II. These include:
- Alteration in breathing patterns, including sleep apnea
- Depressed gag reflex
- Loss of strength in the arms
- Involuntary eye movements that are rapid and downward

In infants, symptoms of a Chiari malformation may include drooling, gagging, a weak cry or irritability when being fed. As the infant grows, they may have developmental disorders and a low weight.

How do I know if my symptoms are caused by a Chiari malformation?

Simply put: you can't. If you have five or more of the above symptoms, it might be a clue that your symptoms *could* be due to a CM. However, those symptoms could easily be caused by one of dozens of other diseases. Complicating the issue is that even if you do have CM, all of your symptoms may not be due to the CM itself. For example, you could have a CM but your headaches could be caused by migraines, sinus issues or stress. That's one of the reasons a CM diagnosis is often hard to come by. If your doctor suspects that CM is the root cause of your symptoms, you'll need extensive testing before the conclusion can be drawn that CM is the actual cause.

My symptoms get worse when I'm ill. Is this normal?

Many people with CM report that their symptoms do get worse when they are ill. However, it can be hard to differentiate between the symptoms being caused by the CM and symptoms that are caused by the illness. It could be that your illness is just adding on some symptoms that make you feel worse. For example, muscle weakness is common with CM, so if you have the flu (which also causes muscle fatigue), you might feel like you've run a marathon. Some patients also report that their symptoms get worse with hot and humid weather, but like most symptoms, this is only a clue.

Keeping a Journal

Unfortunately, many of the symptoms of Chiari can also be caused by other disorders – hundreds of other disorders -- including stress, multiple sclerosis, cluster headaches and even Parkinson's disease. This makes it impossible for you to self-diagnose and it's difficult for any doctor to diagnose the condition. One tool you can use to keep track of your symptoms is a journal. Note your symptoms and how they improve or get worse. You may want to use a scale of 1 to 10 for 1 being mild and 10 for severe. A journal will also help you when you visit the doctor. Often, doctor's visits are rushed (appointments are getting shorter and shorter) and having a journal will help you keep your most important or most severe symptoms at the top of your list.

A great number of Chiari malformations do not produce symptoms and therefore go undiagnosed for a long time. A physical exam can provide clues (such as a balance test or poor reflexes), but usually your physician will order a diagnostic test like a CT scan or an MRI to confirm the diagnosis. This lack of a single diagnostic tool, plus the fact that the wide range of symptoms can also be caused by a huge array of other diseases, sometimes means that CMs are misdiagnosed as another condition like chronic fatigue, migraines, Lou Gehrig's, carpal tunnel and even viruses. Some Chiari patients may go years before getting a firm diagnosis; one study reported that 57% of Chiari patients had their symptoms dismissed as a mental or emotional problem by their physician. In another study of patients diagnosed with fibromyalgia, 46% of patients were shown to have abnormalities in the spinal canal, with 20% having a Type I Chiari malformation. Missed diagnoses and mis-diagnoses are common. Take this story from Stef in Tampa, FL:

"I started getting splitting headaches in my early twenties. The pain was so bad, especially when I coughed or sneezed, that I thought I was going to pass out. My doctor diagnosed cluster headaches, which

seemed to make some sense (what did I know? I just wanted the pain to go away)."

This type of story is a common one heard in Chiari patients who may have gone through years of doctor appointments (and with the condition often worsening) before getting a diagnosis. However, the fault isn't necessarily with the physician – it's often the confusing nature of how Chiari itself presents. Sometimes, your primary care physician may not have heard of Chiari malformation. Or they may not be aware of the usual symptoms for the disease. In most cases, headaches and fatigue can be explained by many other common ailments – like viruses – and a physician will try and rule out those common causes first.

Chiari malformations don't always take years to develop. For some patients – the number approaches 50% -- the onset of symptoms can be quite sudden. This sudden onset of symptoms follows a precipitating event like a fall, accident, infection, or even pregnancy and air travel.

One of the primary tools at a physician's disposal for diagnosing CM is a subjective assessment of a patient's symptoms. The most common symptoms reported are headaches, dizziness, neck pain, insomnia (sleeplessness), fatigue, difficulty swallowing, shortness of breath, nausea, blurred vision and motor problems/strange sensations/numbness in the hands and arms.

Nearly all CM patients suffer from headaches, but as many disorders and diseases can cause headaches, it's often a judgment call on the physician's part as to whether to order additional testing. The headache associated with Chiari is so specific it's often called a "Chiari headache." The headache is a pressure type of ache that starts in the back of the head and may radiate to the front. It's made worse by coughing, sneezing, laughing, bending or straining.

"I had a headache for six months before my diagnosis. The pain (which was excruciating) came and went throughout the day. It was a constant, squeezing pressure at the back, sides and top of my head. My ears felt full (like my sinuses were on fire) and I had a feeling like a piece of beef jerky was lodged in the back of my throat." Sue, Glens Falls NY.

To complicate matters, Chiari headaches and migraines are very closely linked. In fact, it's quite common for the two to be confused, even by physicians. This description of migraines comes from the National Institutes of Health:

"Migraines cause severe pain on one or both sides of the head, upset stomach, and, at times, disturbed vision. People often describe migraine pain as pulsing or throbbing in one area of the head. During migraines, people become very sensitive to

light and sound. They may also become nauseous and vomit."

As you can probably tell, it's impossible for a patient to differentiate between a migraine and a Chiari headache. It's also impossible for a physician to tell the difference just from a physical exam and health history.

CM patients have reported a dizzying array of symptoms, from a hoarse voice to word-finding problems and slurred speech. This isn't surprising, considering the wide range of body functions controlled by the cerebellum. However, it can mean that a diagnosis is difficult to come by. This story, from a Chiari patient, Ted R. is one example of how a CM diagnosis can be a lengthy process:

"I started having some vague symptoms in my early thirties. A throbbing headache in the back of my head that was made worse by coughing, strange aches in my arms and lower back. I put it down to stress. I also had memory issues – I struggled to find words sometimes and joked about how it was my "impending old age." The symptoms ebbed and flowed until my late thirties when the headaches got more frequent and I had weakness in my right leg. It was only to the point of what I would describe as disabling that I went to see my doctor. I only wish I hadn't ignored the symptoms and went a few years earlier."

It's very common for **extremities** (arms, legs) to become affected by CM. Your muscles may become weakened or there may be sensory disturbances (strange sensations in your limbs) including seemingly unexplained pain. The cognitive problems that Ted describes (difficulty finding words) can also be an issue with CM, although cognitive problems can be indicative of dozens of other disorders, including the very common condition of insomnia (inability to sleep). Some CM patients describe a "brain fog" which can also be caused by depression, insomnia, and a variety of disorders either on their own or in combination with CM.

Although not very common, **vestibular testing** can be a strong predictor for CM. Vestibular (balance) problems can originate in the inner ear. Vestibular testing is a non-invasive test where a medical professional will test your balance using a variety of techniques including slowly rotating you on a special chair. The cerebellum sends signals to the inner ear regarding balance, so if the cerebellum is compressed it can affect balance. In a 2002 study, Kumar et al. studied the vestibular testing results for 77 Chiari patients. More than half the group showed abnormal results for the series of 6 tests. In one test that involved irrigating the ears, 75% showed abnormal results.

A condition that often goes along with balance problems is **nystagmus** – a rapid eye movement that often accompanies vertigo (dizziness). As such, CM patients may have nystagmus which may be directly related to Chiari malformation or it may indirectly be related because of the fact that the vertigo might be producing the nystagmus (rather than it being a direct consequence of the malformation itself). Some other eye problems are thought to be connected to CM, including strabismus (sometimes called a lazy eye), a condition where the eyes don't align in synch.

Chiari malformation can cause **breathing problems**, during the day or during sleep. When the breathing difficulties occur during sleep, it is called sleep apnea. It's a condition where you temporarily stop breathing while you are sleeping. Sleep apnea is diagnosed if several events happen where you stop breathing while sleeping, partially wake up and then resume breathing. Sleep apnea is more common in cases of CM where the patient also has syringomyelia (a cavity or cyst in the spinal cord that is filled with CSF fluid). In fact, the number of CM/syringomyelia patients who also have sleep apnea may be as high as 75%.

Although sleep apnea can be a serious condition, in many cases you may not know if you have it. This type of sleep disorder can cause secondary effects, like lethargy and depression, which can be caused by CM even *without* the sleep apnea. If you are diagnosed with sleep apnea, the good news is that decompression surgery is generally effective at curing this particular symptom. Although sleep apnea or daytime breathing difficulties can be distressing, it is extremely rare that sudden respiratory arrest (you stop breathing completely) occurs.

Depression is a serious problem associated with CM. Gretchen W. of Jacksonville FL had this to say about the depression that accompanied her Chiari:

"The terrible depression hit me in waves. It was easy for me to be sucked into the depression as I didn't know whether it was something I could "shake myself out of" or if it was caused by Chiari itself. Plus, I just felt mentally off, like my thoughts wouldn't go in a straight line. At times I was worried if I was just going to slip away and end up in a psych ward, babbling to myself in the corner of a room. I guess it doesn't help I'm mostly at home by myself – the CM has prevented me from working and some days the pain is so unbearable I don't want to leave my bed, let alone my house..."

In 2004, Mueller and Oro found that almost half of symptomatic Chiari patients also had depression. The rate was almost ten times that found in the general population. It is not yet known if the chronic condition and symptoms of Chiari malformation cause the depression (chronic illness and depression have long been linked), or if depression is directly caused by the cerebellum being compressed.

Scoliosis (curvature of the spine) is sometimes accompanied by CM. However, just because a patient has scoliosis does not mean they have CM. In fact, other causes are much more likely to be a cause of scoliosis than CM. If neurological problems are present in addition to CM, it provides one further clue to the diagnosing physician that a CM may be the root cause.

A note on symptoms in children
Although children can experience all of the symptoms associated with CM that adults do, it's thought that oropharyngeal problems (problems with the throat, including choking, chronic cough, and reflux) were the most common symptoms reported in younger children.

Diagnostic tests

Once your doctor suspects Chiari (usually because of your symptoms), they will likely order further testing to help confirm the diagnosis. Some cases of Chiari are easier to diagnose than others. For example, if you have a slew of classic symptoms (like a Chiari headache) and the MRI shows a tonsillar herniation with crowding, it's easier for a physician to diagnose CM as opposed to a list of vaguer symptoms and no crowding on the MRI. A diagnosis is therefore, almost always a judgment call based on the doctor's experience with CM.

The modified Valsalva test

This non-invasive test is performed to find out if your headaches are caused by a tonsillar herniation found on an MRI.

Headaches are a common malady for people even without a CM, and there can be many causes. As one of the primary reasons to undergo surgery is to alleviate disabling symptoms, it's relatively important for your doctor (and you) to know if your symptoms will improve after surgery. If your headaches are caused by something else (like the common migraine), surgery will not improve your headaches.

Sometimes you'll have a "classic" Chiari headache in the back of your head (often described as a disabling, pounding, throbbing ache above your neck). However, everyone is different and it may be that even non-classic headaches are a result of your CM.

The modified Valsalva test involves a Valsalva maneuver, which is where you forcefully attempt to exhale while your airway is closed. This is usually performed while closing your mouth, holding your nose and forcefully breathing out (like you're blowing up a balloon). The modified version may involve breathing out slowly through your teeth although there is no gold standard for how the maneuver is performed. The maneuver has potential risks, like elevating blood pressure. It should **not** be performed at home as it increases your chance of passing out.

MRI

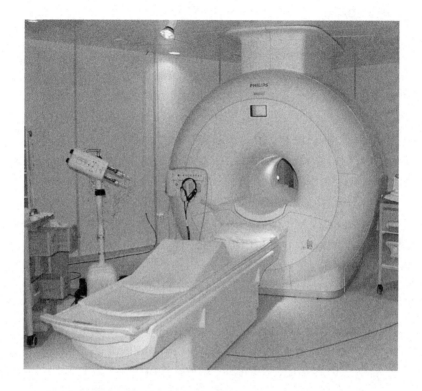

This is the primary test to diagnose CM. An MRI is a safe, painless technique to produce detailed 3-D images of your brain. Although the test is painless, many people feel claustrophobic during the test, as you'll lay on a stretcher in a tube for the procedure. The machine itself is extremely noisy (you'll hear loud, random banging sounds) and takes around 45 minutes to complete – during which time you'll have to lay completely still. You'll be given ear protection and a "panic button" so that you can alert the technician if you have difficulties during the test. If you have an issue with claustrophobia, you can ask your doctor to provide a mild sedative (like Valium) for the procedure.

MRIs are extremely safe, and there are no known side effects from the imaging procedure itself. On the rare occasion the machine does cause harm, it's usually unrelated to the imaging itself. Make sure you tell the technician if you have any metal in your body. You'll be given a comprehensive questionnaire when you arrive for the test which will ask about potential objects that can cause issues – make sure you read it completely. Aneurism clips and pacemakers are just two devices that could cause serious issues. In addition, some MRI accidents have happened because of:

1. Projectiles. The MRI is a giant magnet and on rare occasions, objects have been sucked into the magnetic field. In 2001, a child was killed when an oxygen canister was sucked into the machine.

2. Burns. Don't touch the walls of the MRI tunnel as it carries the risk of severe burns. If there is a risk of you coming into contact with the wall, the technician should place some kind of padding between the patient and the wall. Despite precautions, there have been some cases of burns being so severe that patients have needed skin grafts.

3. Hearing loss. The machines are *very, very* loud. You'll be given hearing protection, so make sure you keep it on at all times when in the room.

Unlike an X-Ray, which cannot show brain tissue, an MRI can show which parts of the brain are protruding into the foramen magnum. There is no connection between how large the malformation is and what your symptoms are or what your prognosis might be – each CM is very individual and affects each person in a different way. For example, if two people have the same size CM where the cerebellar tonsils are protruding by the same amount, one person may have no symptoms at all while the other person might be experiencing severe symptoms. It is mainly for this reason that the MRI is only one tool to confirm a CM diagnosis. It is generally used in combination with a physical exam and neurological exam to classify the severity of the CM and to predict an outcome. It's important to note that unless a radiologist is specifically looking for a Chiari malformation, it may be missed. In fact, one study showed that MRI readings missed 50% of herniations – even with significant CMs of over 5mm.

"It was really tight in the tunnel. So tight that there was only above six inches above my head. But it wasn't as bad as I thought it would be. Both ends were open, so it wasn't quite as claustrophobic as I thought. I was surprised that the table moved – that was a little disconcerting, but the big thing for me is that I had my husband in the room. That made me a bit calmer during the procedure (he could rescue me if I needed!)." Jill—Houston, TX.

Cine-MRI

This test shows the flow of cerebrospinal fluid. It can tell if a Chiari malformation is blocking the flow of CSF, and how much of that blockage is present. Although the technician will use slightly different equipment, from a patient's point of view the experience is the same as having a regular MRI except that you'll have either a wristband or EKG leads on you to monitor your heart rate. These tests are sometimes ordered when your original MRI was "borderline" for Chiari, although they aren't in common use at the time of writing.

Neurological Exam

A neurologist will give you this low-tech test to see how your body reacts to different stimuli and tasks. You may be prodded and poked with a variety of low-tech (and usually, painless) gadgets like hammers, needles and temperature probes. You may be asked to raise your limbs, walk in a straight line, smile, frown or perform a series of manual tasks like touching your thumb to the tips of your fingers.

Brainstem auditory evoked potential (BAER)

An electrical test which examines the function of the hearing apparatus and brainstem connections. This test is used to find out if your brainstem is working properly. The test involves placing electrodes on your scalp and then recording the signals your brain produced in response to auditory stimuli. It is a completely painless procedure.

Computed tomography scan (CT or CAT scan)

A CAT scan is a diagnostic exam similar to x-rays. However, it uses many x-rays to provide a detailed picture of inside the body; it is a good test to define the size of the cerebral ventricles and showing an obvious blockage. The CAT scan machine looks like a large donut. It's an open machine with a much shorter tube that does not have the claustrophobic feel of an MRI.

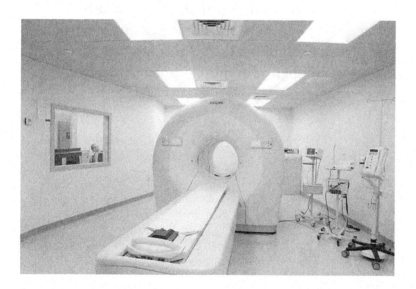

Myelogram
A myelogram uses x-rays in combination with a special dye called a contrast material (a non-toxic dye) to get a detailed picture of the spine and subarachnoid space. The procedure usually involves the injection of the contrast medium into the spine, followed by several X-rays. A numbing agent will be given before

the injection, which should be painless. This is not a common procedure – it has mostly been replaced by CT or MRI scans. However, if you can't have an MRI because of a pacemaker or other implanted object, this test can be used as a replacement.

Somatosensory evoked potential (S SEP)
An S SEP is an electrical test of the nerves involved in sensation, which gives some information about peripheral nerve, spinal cord, and brain function. This is a non-invasive test. A stimulating electrode is placed on your arm or leg, and recording electrodes are placed on your head and/or spine. The test is painless although your muscles may twitch.

Treatment Options

As alarming as the term "Chiari malformation" might be, if your CM is asymptomatic (i.e. it doesn't have any symptoms), the usual course of treatment is to do nothing unless the CM starts to produce symptoms that interfere with your daily living activities.

Unfortunately, there are few treatment options for Chiari malformation outside of surgery. Treatment usually consists of a "wait and see" approach, supplemented with medication to help you manage pain or other symptoms. When your symptoms become intolerable, this is usually the time your doctor will recommend surgery. However, just as there is no golden standard for the diagnosis of CM, there's also no hard and fast rule for when a surgeon will decide to operate. Again, it's usually a judgment call on the part of the neurosurgeon.

In the meantime, medications for certain symptoms (like headaches) may be prescribed. If you have no symptoms at all (for example, if your CM was found incidentally on an MRI), it may be possible that you'll never need surgery. A non-symptomatic CM might just stay exactly the same way over the years. Chiari surgery is major surgery that comes with risks – if you don't have symptoms, it's often not worth the risk. This can be hard to hear – you might feel like you are a ticking time bomb – but be reassured that many, many people with CM never even know they have one, and it may never cause you problems.

What if you *do* have symptoms? Unfortunately, there isn't a consensus on how bad your symptoms should get before surgery is necessary. One factor is quality of life. If your symptoms include severe pain, disabling symptoms (like loss of balance, breathing difficulties or numbness in your extremities) and your symptoms are affecting your day-to-day living, you could be a candidate for surgery.

It's likely that, after a diagnosis of CM, your neurosurgeon will recommend a wait-and-see approach. In fact, you're more likely to **not** have surgery right away; most Chiari patients will not have surgery right after their diagnosis. If you don't have surgery, how closely you are monitored (i.e. how often you have follow-up MRIs), will depend on you, your symptoms, and your physician's judgment. If you have mild symptoms or no symptoms, your doctor may choose to monitor you by regular check-ups and periodic MRI scans. Prescription pain killers or over-the counter drugs may help to control headaches. You should also try to minimize any strain on your neck:

• Ice packs on your neck and shoulders can help relieve pain. Try an actual ice pack for 20 minutes or try an "Icy" product from the pharmacy (found in the pain relief section).

- Sleep on a firm bed with a good pillow and try your best to get at least 8 hours of sleep. If you feel fatigued during the day, ask your doctor about the possibility of sleep apnea or another sleep disorder which may prevent you from getting a good night's sleep.

- Maintain a normal weight. Extra pounds can contribute to leg, back, neck and shoulder pain.

- Drink plenty of water – at least 8 glasses a day.

- Participate in low-impact activities like biking, swimming and walking. Tai Chi or Yoga can help to stretch and tone muscles – they also help to reduce stress. Make sure you speak with your instructor about your CM and avoid yoga poses which might aggravate your symptoms.

- Make sure you wear good, supportive shoes to avoid pounding to your spine and skull.

Avoid these activities

- High-velocity chiropractic manipulation or cervical traction. Chiari patients are cautioned against chiropractics; spinal manipulation cannot "fix" a CM and it may make your condition worse. There have been cases of CM patients deteriorating drastically after chiropracty. If you do want to explore chiropractics or any other alternative medicine, make sure you discuss the plan with your physician before seeking treatment.

- Any sports or other activities that apply G forces to the neck. Examples: roller coasters and other high-velocity thrill rides, high-board diving and scuba diving. You should also avoid contact sports like football or rugby.

- High impact aerobics.

- Any physical activity that puts you at a risk for a fall.

- Heavy lifting (more than 15 pounds) – especially if you have a syrinx.

- Straining on the toilet, which can cause a syrinx to worsen.

A note on pregnancy:

If you are pregnant or are thinking of getting pregnant and you have CM, make sure to discuss your condition with your neurosurgeon and your gynecologist. Some procedure, like epidurals, can be dangerous if you have CM, with or without a syrinx. In addition, the physical force of straining during delivery can cause issues as well. However, with the right precautions it is possible for you to have a completely normal and safe pregnancy.

Are there other options?

Research has been performed regarding the possibility of less invasive treatment procedures since the current methods that are available involve complex, invasive surgeries.

In 2009, a 15 year old boy with type I Chiari Malformation underwent a new, minimally invasive spine surgery procedure that was performed through his nose. The boy had come into the medical center presenting headaches, weakness in the arms, and difficulty in swallowing. He had some speech problems, and he was lacking his gag reflex. Once he was diagnosed with type I Chiari Malformation, the surgeons performed decompression surgery to take pressure off of his brain stem. In order to try and perform this surgery in a less invasive way, the surgeons used the through-the-nose (trans-nasal) approach.

In the trans-nasal approach, an endoscope with a light guide and a very small camera is used and surgical tools can be inserted to do a much less traumatic version of the original surgical procedure. The patient had a good recovery, and a month after the surgery, the symptoms were gone. Although this less invasive procedure had been used in adults in the past, this was the first time that it had been successfully performed on a child. This case showed that this procedure can be a viable alternative for children who suffer this type of malformation. Based on the results, the authors of the research strongly suggest magnetic resonance imaging in all patients with juvenile scoliosis when treatment options like spinal fusion are being considered, especially if it's the case of rapidly progressing scoliosis.

The fact remains though, that for most Chiari patients, the trans-nasal procedure may not be an option.

How to find a Chiari surgeon

There isn't one comprehensive database for Chiari surgeons. Many people use word of mouth (made a lot easier by the number of Chiari-related discussion boards on the web). The "Internet Resources" section of this book also gives you a few places to start with checking credentials. However, you can also consider:

1. Your insurance company. Unfortunately, your choices may be constricted by your insurance company's in-network providers. Ask your insurance company for a list of neurosurgeons. You can also ask about out-of-network costs to possibly use a doctor who isn't in-network. However, seeing as this is major surgery (it can cost anywhere from $30,000 to $150,000 and up depending on what type of surgery you have and what complications may happen) out-of-network is often not an option for most people.

2. Use the AANS site (www.neurosurgerytoday.org) to find board certified neurosurgeons near you.
3. Search your state's Board of Medicine website for malpractice information on any physicians you are considering.
4. Make a shortlist. Ask your insurance company how many neurosurgeons you are allowed to see for opinions and prioritize your list accordingly.

Tip: Call around local hospitals and ask about charitable discounts. Co-pays and deductibles can add up to tens-of-thousands of dollars and many hospitals (Especially those with a religious affiliation) have programs to help low-income patients with treatment.

"I was terrified at the thought of brain surgery, but I needn't have been. A strange, pre-op calmness descended on me (which I'm told is very common). There was some pre-op pain, but the medications I was given in recovery were more than adequate."
Rosalyn, Schenectady, NY.

What Surgery is Like

Surgery to repair a Chiari malformation is called **posterior fossa decompression**. The surgery, performed by a neurosurgeon, creates room around the cerebellar tonsils to ease compression and restore the regular flow of cerebrospinal fluid. The goal of surgery is to ease the pressure and return the tonsils to a normal, rounded shape.

You can expect to spend 3 to 4 hours on the operating table and wake up in the intensive care unit, where you will be closely monitored for 24 hours. The typical patient spends about 2-3 additional days in a recovery ward.

Surgical techniques for CM are constantly being updated, so you would be wise to have any procedure performed by a Chiari malformation specialist, as opposed to a general neurosurgeon. For example, one outdated technique that is sometimes still used is opening the dura and then stitching the edges of the dura to the tissues at the back of the neck. This procedure can cause problems if the meningocele (created during the procedure) doesn't shrink. Most Chiari specialists will use a more modern technique for duraplasty. Ask your neurosurgeon about their experience with Chiari.

Chiari malformation is a major surgery and so you should be prepared for significant pain a long recovery. The back of your head will be shaved to prepare you for the incision (usually a few inches long, from the top of your neck to almost the top of your skull) and you'll be prepared for general anesthesia, including the placement of an IV – an intravenous line, usually into your arm. It's a fairly painless procedure to have an IV inserted; the sensation is very similar to having blood drawn.

You'll be intubated (a breathing tube will be placed down your throat) *after* you are fully anesthetized so you won't be aware of the tube. Your throat may be sore after the surgery. When you are prepared for surgery, your head will be secured with clamps – they will leave post-op marks.

Chiari surgery can take on many forms, depending on the specifics of your condition. For example, the surgery will be different if you need a shunt or spinal stability. This general overview will show you what you can expect from most types of CM surgery. However, you should ask your surgeon what to expect for your specific surgery.

Decompression Surgery

Decompression surgery may involve:

Cranioectomy
The removal of a piece of your skull. Typically, the amount removed will be small (about 3-4cm). This provides decompression and will allow your herniated tonsils to resume a normal shape. The bone may be replaced with a Chiari plate (a metal grid) to re-attach

any muscles that may have been displaced during surgery.

Laminectomy

A procedure to remove the back part of one or more vertebrae to allow decompression. This is usually combined with a cranioectomy. Your surgeon may also remove any scars or adhesions that are present.

Tonsillectomy

Removing all or part of the cerebellar tonsils. This procedure is commonly performed along with a cranioectomy, although in some cases a tonsillectomy is performed without any bone removal. A tonsillectomy may be done with heat, a process called cauterization.

Duraplasty

After bone removal, your surgeon may patch the dura (the protective covering for the brain). Opening the dura can lead to a greater risk of complications (including CFS leaks) and infections. Not all cases of CM surgery require opening of the dura, although it's thought that many unsuccessful surgeries are as a result of the surgeon *not* opening the dura to address issues with CSF flow. Another technique that may be used is **dural scoring** where small incisions are made in the dura (instead of complete removal). On average, you can expect to have a shorter time in the OR and a slightly shorter hospital stay if you have dural scoring instead of duraplasty.

Materials used for duraplasty include a tissue graft from your own body, a tissue graft from a cadaver, bovine (cow) material – taken from the cow's pericardium (heart material), and animal collagen. Synthetic dural grafts are also available. The risks for infection are higher with grafts from a cadaver, which carries a very small risk of the transmission of Creutzfeldt-Jakob disease (CJD), a fatal neurodegenerative disease similar to "Mad Cow Disease". Which graft used is usually up to the surgeon's preference.

At the time of writing, there is a clinical trial underway to find out which types of dural grafts are superior. The Study, run by St. Joseph's Hospital and Medical Center, Phoenix involves surgery and follow-up for 12 months. The study is expected to run through 2018. In order to participate, you must have symptomatic Chiari Malformation described as greater or equal to 6mm descent of the cerebellar tonsils below the foramen magnum with accompanying headaches and/or neurologic findings (arm pain/weakness, myelopathy, etc.). The contacts for the study are:

Justin Clark M.D. 602-746-1468

Ernest Wright M.D. 602-746-0872

Complications

Complication rates for CM are on par with other major surgeries. About 10% of patients experience complications. The rates tend to be higher if the dura is opened. A few reports have shown that the complication rate is zero for surgeries that only involve bony decompressions. Most complications are not life-threatening. The more common complications include: a CSF leak, infection, psuedomeningocele (a bulge in the subarachnoid space, where the CSF circulates), graft issues (inflammation and scarring), and cerebellar slumping (the cerebellum slumps down further after surgery).

General Anesthesia

Chiari malformation surgery is performed under general anesthesia. The anesthesiologist will give you medication in a vein (through an IV) and you may be asked to breathe gas through a mask. During the procedure, your heart rate, breathing ad blood pressure will be closely monitored. You'll also be checked to make sure you are deeply asleep. You won't have any memories of the procedure and you won't feel any pain. You are at a higher risk of complications from general anesthesia if you:

- Abuse alcohol or medications
- Have allergies or a family history of being allergic to medicine
- Have heart, lung, or kidney problems

- Are a smoker
- Have sleep apnea
- Are obese
- Have diabetes, high blood pressure or other medical conditions that affect your heart, kidneys or lungs
- Are an older adult

Complications include:

- Death (rare, about 1 in 100,000 to 1 in 200,000)
- Stroke (rare)
- Temporary mental confusion (rare)
- Waking during anesthesia (rare, thought to be about 1 or 2 in 1,000)
- Harm to your vocal cords
- Hypothermia
- Hypoxic brain damage
- Embolism
- Backache
- Heart attack
- Lung infection
- Mental confusion (temporary)
- Stroke
- Trauma to your teeth or tongue (about 1 in 4,500)
- Nausea (about 30% of patients)

The thought of waking up during surgery (unintended intraoperative awareness) and feeling pain can be terrifying, but it happens rarely. It's more common in people who use alcohol daily, are depressed, or have heart or lung problems.

What you'll feel like after surgery

After surgery, you'll probably wake up in a recovery room where your vital signs will be closely monitored. Your level of consciousness, arm and leg strength, breathing, heart rate and blood pressure will all be monitored. You'll be closely monitored (likely in an ICU) for 24 hours after surgery. This is the period that poses the greatest risk for post-op bleeding.

Although you won't feel pain during surgery, CM surgery is a major procedure and you will feel some pain afterwards. It can take time for the muscles and other tissues to heal after the operation. You'll be asked not to move for the first day or so, then gradually you'll be eased back into your daily living activities. A dull headache is very common after a CM procedure. Most CM patients will experience a lot of neck pain and stiffness in the first few days after a CM decompression due to the displacement of neck muscles during surgery. You'll be given pain medication to help you through the post-op days.

It's common to feel fatigue after any operation. This can be due to a combination of factors, including the physical stress of the surgery itself or even anxiety leading up to the procedure. Depending on how involved your surgery was, it's likely to take a few months to a year to fully recover. Many Chiari patients report that they feel weak for up to 3 months after the operation. A very gradual return to normal activities combined with lots of rest is advisable. Some aches and pains can be expected after surgery, but **you should call your doctor (or go to the ER) immediately if you have a stiff neck with: nausea and dizziness, an intense headache, or a high fever.** This could be a sign of a CSF leak or an infection.

In general, you can expect to experience the following symptoms after the operation. These are considered normal symptoms and usually don't mean that anything is seriously wrong:

- Daily headaches that may last for a few weeks. As you heal, these should become less frequent.
- Neck pain, which is the most common symptom.
- Numbness in the skull from where your skin nerves were cut. Although this will gradually get better, you may always have a little numbness in this area.
- Impaired concentration that may last for weeks or months.
- Irritability, depression, crying spells, and anxiety are also common after a surgery.

- Tiredness and fatigue, which will gradually improve.

Your incision will be covered by a dressing. This will probably be checked and re-dressed a few days after your surgery. You should keep the wound dry for at least two weeks after. If you have staples, they will be removed after about a week. Although you can resume a moderate exercise regime (i.e. walking an hour a day) after surgery, you should not drive or operate heavy machinery until you have the go ahead from your surgeon. Avoid hair color, perms, hair mouse or gel for at least 2 months post-op. You should also avoid running or riding bicycles for at least two months. You can have sex, but don't participate in very rigorous sexual activity for at least a month post-op.

Surgery under general anesthesia is thought to affect cognitive function and declines in cognitive ability have been found after surgery. You may experience problems like a lack of concentration and attention. This is much more likely to happen if you are an older adult. About 25% of those over 60 years-old will experience cognitive problems, which is usually temporary. You will probably be back to normal in a few weeks.

"I went though physical therapy after my op to learn to walk properly again as prior to the surgery I'd had significant balance problems and a limp. Post-surgery, the pain disappeared but I still had some

numbness which I was told would never heal (it was caused by nerve damage). It took about 6 months to feel like I was back to my old self but it did take a couple of years before I could return to my old teaching job. The pain did slowly return, but it's manageable with meds." Sam, Dallas TX.

Preoperative safety steps

Make sure you have a complete and thorough preoperative discussion with the anesthesiologist before your surgery. Make sure you fill out a complete medical history questionnaire. Of particular importance is any adverse reactions to anesthesia in yourself or your parents, siblings, or children. Bring a list of all medications you take (including over the counter drugs, like aspirin or St. John's Wort).

The preoperative interview is also a good time to find out what anesthetic will be used during surgery and what side effects you are likely to experience.

Other Surgery Types

The gold standard for CM surgery is decompression surgery. However, if you have other issues, you may need other surgeries. These can include:

- The implantation of a shunt to redirect the flow of CSF. Used when you have excess CSF in the brain (a condition called hydrocephalus) or hypertension (elevated pressure in the brain).

- Fusion or stabilization may be used to stabilize your neck in cases where you have an extensive laminectomy or you need more support for your head.

Surgery Outcomes

As there are many types of CM surgery that come with many possible add-on conditions (like spina bifida), it's impossible to predict which patients will fully recover from symptoms after a CM surgery. In general, you have about a 30% to 50% chance of becoming completely symptom free after surgery. Thirty percent of post-op patients will have significant improvements in symptoms and their quality of life. In other words, between 60% and 80% of surgeries are a "success." If you have moderate to severe blockage of CSF, you are more likely to have a successful surgery. If you have a frontal headache (as opposed to the classic Chiari headache at the back of your skull), you are much less likely (about four times less likely) of having a "successful" surgery. Patients who also had scoliosis were nine times likely to have a poor surgical outcome.

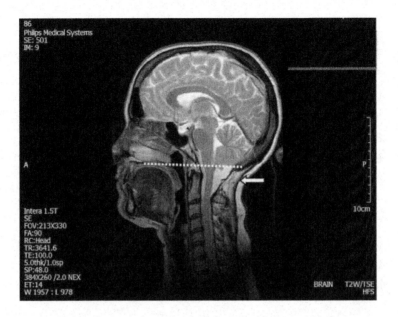

Post surgery: The occipital craniectomy scar (the white arrow to the right) and tonsillar upward migration above hard plate-foramen magnum line (the dotted white line). In other words, this picture shows that post-surgery, the cerebellar tonsils have returned to a normal position and are no longer herniated.

Alternative Treatments

There are no alternative treatments that can treat CM. However, acupuncture may help with the pain. Acupuncture is a family of procedures that involve stimulating anatomical points on your body using a variety of techniques. In most cases, acupuncture normally means that your skin will be penetrated with thin, solid, metallic needles that are manipulated by a practitioner's hands or by electrical stimulation. Acupuncture is a key component of traditional Chinese medicine, but it is also widely practiced in the United States. According to the 2007 National Health Interview Survey, which included a comprehensive survey of complementary and alternative medicine use by Americans, an estimated 3.1 million U.S. adults and 150,000 children had used acupuncture in the previous year.

Acupuncture is a very safe procedure that is regulated by The U.S. Food and Drug Administration (FDA). For example, the FDA requires that any needles used in the procedure are sterile, nontoxic, and labeled for single use by qualified practitioners.

There are no current studies that show acupuncture is effective to control the pain associated with any chronic condition, including CM. Whether it's a placebo effect or if the procedure actually does stimulate the brain to produce less of the signals that transmit pain is not fully understood. However, many patients report that it does help.

"I had tried just about everything for the headaches, including several prescriptions from my physician. A friend recommended an acupuncturist and I thought – what have I got to lose? The doctor spent about an hour asking me about my symptoms and then spent some time mapping out where he was going to place the needles (I think he used some kind of special marker on my back for this, but I can't be sure). The insertion of the needles was relatively

painless – kind of like being flicked by a finger. Then he left the room for ten minutes and came back, asked me how I felt. I didn't feel any different, honestly, so he said he would give it another ten minutes. The second time he came back in I realized that the pain had gone! I was completely astounded – I never expected it to work that well. I now go back for monthly treatments. It definitely reduces the pain to a very manageable level and a lot of the time I have no headache at all." Ellen, Topeka KS.

If you decide to try acupuncture, make sure to check any practitioner's credentials. Most states require acupuncturists to be licensed (see the Resources section at the back of this book for information on state licensing).

Prognosis

As we've stated before, how successful your surgery is depends on what other related conditions you have, your overall health and other factors.

If your only condition is Chiari malformation (i.e. you do not have secondary conditions like spina bifida or syringomyelia), and you have successful surgery, you have about an 80% chance of a positive outcome where your symptoms are reduced to only a few symptoms or none at all. Twenty percent of patients will not see any improvement, or will see their condition worsen. Some of these patients have other conditions, like Pseudotumor cerebri.

A review of 192 patients who had undergone posterior fossa decompression showed that 36 of these 192 patients hadn't shown any improvement during a follow up period of up to 6 years post-surgery. A large percentage of the patients who showed post-operative symptoms had Type I Chiari

Malformation and Pseudo-Tumor Cerebri -- high cerebrospinal fluid pressure in the head -- with no apparent cause. The symptoms of these patients varied, but most of them presented head pain of some sort. The studies showed that the surgical intervention itself could have caused changes in the flow of cerebrospinal fluid, which in turn could lead to the development of PTC after the surgery. So, it was concluded that in the cases of decompression surgery involving complications caused by increased intracranial pressure, additional procedures involving the drainage of cerebrospinal fluid should be taken into consideration. In addition, the study showed that evaluating patients for high cerebrospinal fluid pressure before decompression surgery can also be of great value in assessing the chances of a positive surgical outcome.

In general (and assuming you don't have any other conditions), the less time you have had symptoms, the better your chances are of a good outcome from surgery. In addition, patients who have a severe blockage of cerebrospinular fluid usually have better outcomes than patients who have mild blockages. How well you recover from surgery can also depend on your overall physical health, how much time you can afford to spend on your recovery (in other words, people who take a few weeks off work generally do better than those who have to rush back to the job) and what complications (if any) presented during surgery. You will probably rest at home for up to 6 weeks, followed by a gradual return to your normal activities. You can expect a full recovery in about 3 to 4 months. If you have had surgery for syringomyelia, your recovery may take longer – up to a year or more.

Can I Die from Chiari Malformation?

As distressing as the disorder is, Chiari malformation rarely leads to death and is not considered to be a terminal illness or disease. However, there have been some reports in the medical literature of CM-related deaths, including several cases of sudden respiratory arrest and minor trauma to the head that resulted in death (Chiari malformations were found on autopsy). These sudden deaths are likely related to a malfunctioning brain stem and are very rare cases.

Chiari malformation can be a chronic condition that can lead to other health problems like obesity and depression. These health problems are far more likely to shorten a CM patient's life span than a CM alone.

Can a Chiari Malformation Improve without Surgery?

If you're feeling hesitant about surgery, you may be wondering how long it will be before your symptoms get a lot worse (the answer is, no one knows), or if a CM can "go away" on its own. There *is* a possibility that the CM will disappear and that the cerebellum will return to normal (a condition called spontaneous resolution), but this is a long shot; only a few cases of spontaneous resolution have ever been reported in the medical journals. Of those cases, most were related to syringomyelia, trauma, multiple sclerosis or syrinxes of unknown origin.

Will my Symptoms Come Back?

Even with a successful surgery, there is a chance that your symptoms may come back. There isn't any good data to suggest how often this happens. Several factors can make it much more likely for your symptoms to recur, including trauma. For example, if you have a head injury it could mean that your symptoms might recur. If you keep yourself in good physical health and avoid falls and accidents as much as possible, you're less likely to experience recurring symptoms.

Related Disorders

There are a lot of diseases associated Chiari malformations. Some of the diseases have a very strong relationship – for example, Spina Bifida. According to the Spina Bifida Association, some degree of Chiari malformation is present in the vast majority of people with Spina Bifida, it is thought to be symptomatic in about one of three individuals. Other diseases aren't closely linked, or at least *how* they may be linked isn't fully understood. Even the exact mechanism by which Chiari malformation is formed is subject to debate – which is one reason why there is a lot of research into other disorders. Researchers hope to find links between the disorders and therefore find the underlying mechanisms as to why some people get the disorders and why some people don't. This chapter covers some of the more common disorders known to be linked to Chiari malformation.

The primary link between all of these disorders is a deformation of the posterior cranial fossa. Some of the disorders are congenital and others are thought to be acquired (i.e. due to trauma).

Ehlers-Danlos Syndrome
It is thought that between 1% and 5% of patients may have this condition.

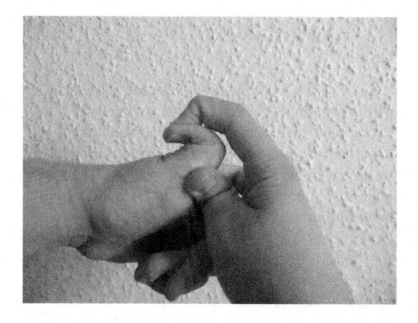

Ehlers-Danlos syndrome is a group of disorders that affect your connective tissues. The connective tissues support the skin, bones, blood vessels, and other organs. If you have EDS, defects in the connective tissues can cause a variety of signs and symptoms ranging from loose joints to life-threatening complications.

There are six major types of EDS:

The arthrochalasia type

The classic type

The dermatosparaxis type

The hypermobility type

The kyphoscoliosis type

The vascular type

All types affect the joints, giving the EDS patient hypermobility of the joints. Some affect the skin. In infants, sitting, standing, and walking may all be delayed. EDS patients are prone to dislocated joints, chronic pain, and early-onset arthritis.

Many people with EDS people have fragile, stretchy skin that has a velvet-like texture. Some individuals may bruise or scar easily. Some forms of EDS can involve serious and potentially life-threatening complications such as blood vessels that can tear unpredictably, causing internal bleeding, stroke, and shock. An increased risk of organ rupture is found with the vascular type of EDS. This can include tearing of the intestine and rupture of the uterus (womb) during pregnancy.

It's thought that about 1 in 5,000 individuals worldwide have EDS. It is genetic, meaning that it's passed down through generations.

Fibromylagia

Fibromyalgia causes muscle pain and fatigue. It may also cause insomnia, morning stiffness, headaches, painful periods, tingling or numbness in the hands and feet and "brain fog" or difficulty with concentration. The disorder is characterized by tender points on the neck, shoulders, back, hips, arms, and legs.

Symptoms of Chiari malformation and fibromyalgia are closely linked. According to the National Fibromyalgia association, this list of symptoms is found in **both** CM and Fibromyalgia:

- Fatigue
- Sleep disturbances
- Impaired memory/concentration
- Nervousness
- Depression
- Leg cramps
- Disorientation
- Word finding difficulty
- Headache at lower back of head, or face
- Migraine
- Neck pain
- Chest pain

- Back pain
- Shoulder pain
- Burning sensations or sensations of small crawling insects on the skin, burning sensations
- Slight eye paralysis of the sixth nerve
- Dry eyes
- Double or blurred vision
- Nystagmus
- Hearing loss, tinnitus, vertigo and other ear problems
- Imbalance
- Dizziness
- Nausea and vomiting
- Fainting
- Low blood pressure
- Lethargy
- Difficulty swallowing
- Upper extremity weakness and numbness
- Lower extremity weakness and numbness
- Stiffness
- Bowel dysfunction
- Incontinence
- Frequent urination
- Sexual dysfunction
- Feeling of stiffness
- Feeling of tightness
- Feeling that your legs are about to collapse

In addition, fibromyalgia symptoms (like Chiari malformation symptoms) can be precipitated by physical trauma, whiplash or surgery. Symptoms in both disorders can worsen with exertion.

A rheumatologist can check for fibromyalgia by figuring out if you have the tender points associated with the disorder, and an MRI can rule out (or in) Chiari malformation.

Interestingly, one study found that 20% of fibromyalgia patients had CM Type 1, with a tonsillar ectopia of greater than 5mm. Many other fibromyalgia patients were found to have a condition related to compression on the spinal cord. What this means for Chiari malformation patients is that many were (incorrectly) diagnosed with fibromyalgia before arriving at a CM diagnosis as the symptoms are so similar. Therefore, it's recommended that fibromyalgia patients are tested for the presence of CM. If you already have a CM diagnosis, it's unlikely (although not impossible) that you also have fibromyalgia.

Hydrocephalus

Hydrocephalus is an excess buildup of cerebrospinal fluid in the brain due to overproduction of CSF or lack of absorption of CSF. The increased fluid causes pressure inside the skull and the bones expand out to make the head appear larger than normal. This condition is commonly seen in Type II CM although it is sometimes seen in children with Type I. Hydrocephalus is found in around 4% to 18% of patients with CM Type I. Severe hydrocephalus can be fatal. For more information, visit the Hydrocephalus Association's website at http://www.Hydroassoc.org.

Craniosynostosis

Craniosynostosis is a birth defect where one or more of the joints in an infant's skull close prematurely, before the brain is fully formed. When an infant has craniosynostosis, their brain is constricted and can't grow in its natural shape. Craniosynostosis and Chiari malformation is strongly associated Craniosynostosis usually happens when the lambdoid sutures (a fibrous connective tissue that connects the parietal bones to the occipital bone) fuse too early in the development of the skull. Chiari malformation is thought to be associated with several forms of craniosynostosis, which may not be present at birth. However once the lambdoid suture fuses, a Chiari malformation may be formed.

Endocrinopathy

Growth hormone deficiency has been linked to Chiari malformation. In fact, CM Type I is seen in about 5%–20% of patients with growth hormone deficiency. The deficiency in growth hormone is thought to be responsible for insufficient development of the posterior fossa. This results in tonsillar herniation.

Hyperostosis

Hyperostosis (excessive growth or thickening of bone tissue) is another condition that can affect the development of the skill. When hyperostosis affects the posterior fossa, it can often result in Chiari malformation. Other, rarer types of hyperostosis that can lead to CM are craniometaphyseal dysplasia (a rare condition characterized by thickening of bones in the skull and abnormalities at the ends of long bones in the limbs), osteopetrosis (also a rare condition, where the bones are abnormally dense) and erythroid hyperplasia (an excessive amount of red blood cell precursors in the bone marrow).

Bone Mineral Deficiency

Patients with hereditary vitamin D–resistant rickets have higher rates of CM Type I. This is thought to be due to the overcrowding of the posterior fossa.

Cutaneous Disorders

Cutaneous disorders occur quite often with CM Type I, although there doesn't seem to a strong link between the two. For example, up to 8% of patients with neurofibromatosis Type I also have CM Type I. Many other cutaneous disorders have been linked with CM Type I, although it could be merely due to coincidence. These include:

- Multiple lentigines syndrome, which is characterized by associated brown skin spots called lentigines that are similar to freckles. The condition has many additional characteristic features including abnormalities in the electrical signals that control the heartbeat and widely spaced eyes.

- Blue rubber bleb nevus syndrome, a condition where there are malformations of the venous system.

- Giant congenital melanocytic nevi – a disorder where there is a nevi (similar to a birthmark or mole) that covers a very large part of the body.

Spinal Defects

Although many causes of Chiari malformation are linked to the posterior fossa and base of the skull, a few other disorders that involve defects of the spine have also been linked to CM Type I. For example, up to 6% of lipomeningomyelocele patients have CM Type I. *Spinal curvature* is common among patients with CM Type I. This includes scoliosis, where the spine bends to the right or left, and kyphosis, where the spine bends forward.

Tethered cord syndrome is another condition closely linked to CM. TCS happens when the spinal cord attaches itself to actual bones of the spine. This causes the spine to stretch, which can result in permanent nerve damage.

Space-occupying Lesions

Lesions in the brain and cerebrospinal fluid leaks (both acquired conditions) are thought to be linked to the development of CM Type I. Lesions and CSF links can be caused by a wide range of conditions, including brain tumors and hematomas (a collection of blood outside of the blood vessels).

Pseudotumor Cerebri

Pseudotumor Cerebri occurs when too much pressure builds up inside the skull. The condition's symptoms are as if the patient had a tumor, but no tumor is present. There is a fairly strong link between pseudotumor cerebri and Chiari Type I. According to Johnston et. Al, 6% of adult pseudotumor cerebri patients also have Chiari malformation type I. The actual mechanism for the connection is unknown.

Spina bifida

Thirty percent of children born with spina bifida also have a CM. Some children with spina bifida have cognitive impairment which is usually attributed to hydrocephalus (excessive cerebrospinal fluid in the brain). However, some research suggests that CM may be responsible for some cognitive impairment, especially with Type II. The link between CM and cognitive impairment is only suggested – it has not been proved. However, it is possible that cognitive impairment is possible in cases of CM Type II *without* the accompanying Spina Bifida. Further research is needed before any conclusions can be drawn.

Syringomyelia / Hydromyelia

Some people with CM (thought to be anywhere from 20% to 70% of patients) will develop this fluid-filled cyst in the spinal cord. Doctors do not know who will develop this condition and who will not. In addition, *why* it occurs in CM is hotly debated. There are, however, many theories including the "piston theory". In the piston theory, it's thought that the cerebellar tonsils act like a piston, creating waves of pressure down the spinal cord with every heartbeat. This forces the cerebrospinal fluid into a sac. Symptoms include weakness and pain in the upper back, neck, shoulders, arms and legs, abnormal sensations, disruptions to sensing hot and/or cold, bladder and/or bowel issues, and abnormal sweating. In severe cases, the cyst can expand, damaging the spinal cord and leading to nerve damage and paralysis.

When syringomyelia is contained within the central canal in the spinal cord, it's sometimes called **hydromyelia**. Symptoms can be similar to Chiari malformation symptoms, although some symptoms tend to occur more if you have this condition:

- Scoliosis
- Loss of sensitivity, especially to hot and cold
- Muscle weakness and spasticity
- Loss of bowel and bladder control
- Motor impairment
- Chronic pain
- Headaches (often concurrent with the Chiari malformation)

Glossary

Arachnoid – see meninges
Atlas -- The first vertebrae. Carries the weight of the head and is a ring-like structure.
Axis is the second vertebrae down; it's the pivot on which the atlas rotates.
Brainstem auditory evoked potential (BAER): An electrical test which examines the function of the hearing apparatus and brainstem connections.
Brainstem -- The part of the brain where the spinal cord connects. It includes the midbrain, pons and medulla.
Central canal – the center of the spinal cord.
Cerebellar ectopia -- where the cerebellum is out of position (not protruding).

Cerebellar hemisphere -- The lateral (side) portion of the cerebellum. This part is primarily involved in body movements, including fine motor movements.
Cerebellar herniation -- When the cerebellum passes through the foramen magnum.
Cerebellar tonsils are located on the underside of the cerebellum. The cerebellar tonsils are thought to influence limb movement and posture.
Cerebellar vermis -- the nerve tissue that connects the two halves of the cerebellum (the part of the brain affected by CM). It regulates the muscles and influences attention, sensation, motivation, memory, behavior and autonomic activities like breathing, digestion and heart rate.
Cerebellum – part of the brain found at the base of the skill.
Cerebrospinal fluid (CSF) is a clear fluid that bathes and protects the brain and spine. It gives a mechanical and immunological protection to the brain and provides a vital role in cerebral blood flow.
Cervical – upper part of the spine (the neck area).
Cervical spina bifida occulta -- a bony defect in the rear part of the spine.
Chiari headache. The headache is a pressure type of ache that starts in the back of the head and may radiate to the front. It's made worse by coughing, sneezing, laughing, bending or straining.
Chiari malformation Type 0 -- A type of CM that produced symptoms. However, the cerebellum is in a normal position.

Chiari malformation Type I -- The lower part of the cerebellum protrudes into the foramen magnum. No symptoms may be present.

Chiari malformation Type II -- The cerebellum and brain stem tissue protrude into the foramen magnum. This type is seen almost exclusively in patients with myelomeningocele, the most common type of spina bifida.

Chiari malformation Type III --The cerebellum and brain stem protrude into the foramen magnum. Part of the fourth ventricle – a fluid-filled cavity in the brain that circulates cerebrospinal fluid -- may also protrude.

Chiari malformation Type IV -- A rare form of CM that involves an underdeveloped or incomplete cerebellum.

Cine-MRI This test shows the flow of cerebrospinal fluid. It can tell if a Chiari malformation is blocking the flow of CSF, and how much of that blockage is present.

Cluster headaches – one of the most painful types of headache, where the headaches occur in cyclical patterns (clusters).

CM – Chiari malformation.

Computed tomography scan (CT or CAT scan) A diagnostic similar to an x-rays. However, it uses many x-rays to provide a detailed picture of inside the body; it is a good test to define the size of the cerebral ventricles and showing an obvious blockage.

Conus medullaris. The conus medullaris is the tapered, lower end of the spinal cord.

Cranioectomy The removal of a piece of your skull.
Cranio vertebral junction – the area where the spine meets the skull.
Craniosynostosis is a birth defect where one or more of the joints in an infant's skull close prematurely, before the brain is fully formed.
Cranium – the skull.
CSF – Cerebospinal fluid.
Decompression surgery – surgery to create space around a CM.
Dura – outer covering of the brain.
Dural scoring where small incisions are made in the dura (instead of complete removal).
Duraplasty After bone removal, your surgeon may patch the dura (the protective covering for the brain).
Ehlers-Danlos syndrome is a group of disorders that affect your connective tissues. The connective tissues support the skin, bones, blood vessels, and other organs.
Embolism – from the Greek "stopper" or "plug", an embolism is where a blood clot (or sometimes a fat globule or gas bubble) lodges in the bloodstream.
Endocrinopathy a disease of the endocrine system, sometimes called a "hormone imbalance" or Growth hormone deficiency.
Fatigue – a feeling of being tired or needing to rest due to lack of strength or energy.
Fibromyalgia is an auto-immune disorder characterized by causes muscle pain and fatigue. It may also cause insomnia, morning stiffness, headaches, painful periods, tingling or numbness in

the hands and feet and "brain fog" or difficulty with concentration.
Foramen magnum, the space in the skull which allows the spinal cord to pass through into the brain.
Fourth ventricle -- a cerebrospinal fluid filled space located behind the brainstem and just in front of the cerebellum.
Genetic -- passed down through generations by genes.
Graft – Tissue surgically implanted to repair or replace a defect.
Hernia – where a part of the body protrudes out of the cavity where it's supposed to be.
Hydrocephalus is an excess buildup of cerebrospinal fluid in the brain due to overproduction of CSF or lack of absorption of CSF.
Hydromyelia when syringomyelia is contained within the central canal in the spinal cord, it's sometimes called hydromyelia.
Hyperostosis -- excessive growth or thickening of bone tissue.
Hypothermia – a condition where your body temperature drops below the normal temperature required for your body to function properly.
Hypoxic brain damage – brain damage caused by a lack of oxygen.
Intracranial pressure (ICP) – buildup of pressure in the skull caused by too much CSF.
Incontinence – involuntary excretion of urine (inability to control your bladder).

Intubated – where a breathing tube is placed down your throat.
Kyphosis is a condition where the spine bends forward.
Lambdoid sutures are (a fibrous connective tissue that connect the parietal bones to the occipital bone.
Laminectomy A procedure to remove the back part of one or more vertebrae to allow decompression.
Lethargy – a state of being abnormally drowsy.
Medulla is a part of the brainstem that contains the cardiac, respiratory, vomiting and vasomotor centers and is associated with breathing, heart rate and blood pressure.
Meninges are a protective layer for the brain and spine. CSF is located in the space between two layers of this protective layer called the arachnoid and the pia mater.
Midbrain is a part of the brainstem associated with vision, hearing, motor control, sleep/wake, arousal (alertness), and temperature regulation.
Migraines *cause severe pain on one or both sides of the head, upset stomach, and, at times, disturbed vision.*
Modified Valsalva test involves a Valsalva maneuver, which is where you forcefully attempt to exhale while your airway is closed.
MRI is a safe, painless technique to produce detailed 3-D images of your brain.
Myelogram -- uses x-rays in combination with a special dye called a contrast material to get a detailed picture of the spine and subarachnoid space. The

procedure usually involves the injection of a contrast medium (a dye) into the spine, followed by several X-rays.

Neurological Exam a low-tech test to see how your body reacts to different stimuli and tasks. You may be prodded and poked with a variety of low-tech (and usually, painless) gadgets like hammers, needles and temperature probes.

Nystagmus – involuntary, rapid eye movement.

Occipital bone -- the bone that covers the cerebellum.

Odontoid process -- the joint between the atlas and the axis.

Oropharyngeal dysfunction is a difficulty with chewing and swallowing.

Oropharyngeal problems (problems with the throat, including choking, chronic cough, and reflux) **Scoliosis** (curvature of the spine.

Perivascular spaces The spaces in the spine where the blood vessels are located.

Pia mater. – see meninges.

Pons is a part of the brainstem associated with sleep, respiration, swallowing, bladder control, hearing, equilibrium, taste, eye movement, facial expressions, facial sensation, and posture.

Posterior fossa decompression -- Surgery to repair a Chiari malformation.

Posterior fossa -- houses the cerebellum.

Pseudotumor Cerebri occurs when too much pressure builds up inside the skull. The condition's symptoms are as if the patient had a tumor, but no tumor is present

Psuedomeningocele -- a bulge in the subarachnoid space, where the CSF circulates.

Sleep apnea is a condition diagnosed if several events happen where you stop breathing while sleeping, partially wake up and then resume breathing.

Extremities – arms and legs.

Somatosensory evoked potential (S SEP): An electrical test of the nerves involved in sensation, which gives some information about peripheral nerve, spinal cord, and brain function.

Spina bifida – a birth defect caused by incomplete closing of the spine around the spinal cord.

Syringomyelia -- forces the cerebrospinal fluid into a sac.

Syrinx – a CSF filled sac.

Tonsillar ectopia -- When the tonsils are out of position (and not protruding).

Tonsillar herniation -- When the cerebellar tonsils protrude through the posterior fossa.

Tonsillectomy Removing all or part of the cerebellar tonsils.

Unintended intraoperative awareness -- waking up during surgery.

Vestibular testing is a non-invasive test where a medical professional will test your balance by asking you to perform some simple maneuvers, like walking with your eyes closed.

Chiari Malformation Organizations

March of Dimes
1275 Mamaroneck Avenue
White Plains, NY 10605
askus@marchofdimes.com
http://www.marchofdimes.com
Tel: 914-997-4488 888-MODIMES (663-4637)
Fax: 914-428-8203

National Organization for Rare Disorders (NORD)
55 Kenosia Avenue
Danbury, CT 06810
orphan@rarediseases.org
http://www.rarediseases.org
Tel: 203-744-0100 Voice Mail 800-999-NORD (6673)
Fax: 203-798-2291

Spina Bifida Association
4590 MacArthur Blvd. NW
Suite 250
Washington, DC 20007-4266
sbaa@sbaa.org
http://www.spinabifidaassociation.org
Tel: 202-944-3285 800-621-3141
Fax: 202-944-3295

American Syringomyelia & Chiari Alliance Project (ASAP)
P.O. Box 1586
Longview, TX 75606-1586
info@asap.org
http://www.asap.org
Tel: 903-236-7079 800-ASAP-282 (272-7282)
Fax: 903-757-7456

Chiari & Syringomyelia Foundation
29 Crest Loop
Staten Island, NY 10312
info@CSFinfo.org
http://www.csfinfo.org
Tel: 718-966-2593
Fax: 718-966-2593 (Call First)

Internet Resources

Merck Manual of Diagnosis and Therapy, 17th ed.

http://www.merck.com/mmpe/index.html

A medical guide for professionals, available online. Contains technical information for a host of diseases along with their corresponding diagnosis and treatment suggestions.

Merck Manual of Medical Information - 2nd Home Edition

http://www.merck.com/mmhe/index.html
A consumers' guide to diseases and their treatments. This is a complete online version of the text edition, with videos and a pronunciation guide

MEDLINE/MedlinePlus

http://www.nlm.nih.gov/medlineplus/

Anatomy videos aimed at the general consumer plus thousands of articles on a variety of health related topics.

PubMed

http://www.ncbi.nlm.nih.gov/sites/entrez
PubMed comprises more than 20 million citations for biomedical literature from MEDLINE, life science journals, and online books. Citations may include links to full-text content from PubMed Central and publisher web sites.

Deciphering Medspeak

http://mlanet.org/resources/medspeak/index.html

To make informed health decisions, you have probably read a newspaper or magazine article, tuned into a radio or television program, or searched the Internet to find answers to health questions. If so, you have probably encountered "medspeak," the specialized language of health professionals. The Medical Library Association developed "Deciphering Medspeak" to help translate common "medspeak" terms.

Alternative Medicine Homepage

http://www.pitt.edu/~cbw/altm.html
From the Falk Library of the Health Sciences, University of Pittsburgh - a jumpstation for sources of information on unconventional, alternative, complementary, innovative, and integrative therapies.

National Center for Complementary and Alternative Medicine

http://nccam.nih.gov/

General information about alternative and complementary therapies with links to research studies currently being conducted on alternative therapies for a variety of conditions.

Rosenthal Center for Complementary and Alternative Medicine

http://www.rosenthal.hs.columbia.edu//

Links to resources on acupuncture, homeopathy, chiropractic, and herbal medicine and alternative therapies for cancer and women's health. The Center sponsors research on alternative and complementary medical practices.

CLINICAL RESEARCH TRIALS

Center Watch

http://www.centerwatch.com/

Information on over 41,000 clinical trials for twenty disease categories. Profiles of 150 research centers conducting clinical trials and profiles of companies that provide a variety of contract services to the clinical trials industry. Includes industry and government sponsored clinical trials and information on new drug treatments approved by the Food and Drug Administration.

Clinical Trials

http://www.clinicaltrials.gov/

Information on current research being conducted on treatments for different diseases. Browse by disease category and sponsor or search the entire site. Learn what clinical trials are all about and how to decide to participate in a trial.

National Organization for Rare Diseases

http://www.rarediseases.org/

Basic information on rare diseases and disorders. Full-reports are available for a fee.

HEALTH CARE PROVIDERS

American Board of Medical Specialties (ABMS)

http://www.abms.org/

Verify the certification status of any physician in the 24 specialties of the ABMS. Registration is required (free) and user is limited to five searches in a 24 hour period.

AMA Physician Select

https://extapps.ama-assn.org/doctorfinder/recaptcha.jsp

Gives credentials of MD's and DO's including medical school, year of graduation, and specialties.

American Hospital Directory

http://www.ahd.com/
Profiles of U.S. hospitals. Basic service is free; more detailed information by paid subscription only.

Federation of State Medical Boards

http://www.fsmb.org/

Select "Public Services" from the left-hand index, then select "Directory of State Medical Boards" to find links to web sites for the 50 U.S. States, plus the District of Columbia, Guam, and the Northern Mariana Islands. Not all of the states have physician profile or disciplinary action information. There are also links to osteopathic physician sites when available.

Health Pages

http://www.healthpages.com/

Information about physicians, dentists, hospitals and clinics, elder care facilities, dietitians and nutritionists.

Joint Commission on the Accreditation of Healthcare Organizations

http://www.jointcommission.org/
The Quality Check feature on this site supplies details on individual hospital performance ratings from JCAHO's accreditation reports. View Performance Reports and compare institutions' ratings. Reports cover hospitals, nursing homes, ambulatory care facilities, home care, laboratory services, and long term care facilities.

Quackery and Health Fraud

Quackwatch

http://www.quackwatch.com/

Want information about whether those alternative therapies work? This site has information on health fraud, medical quackery, "new age" medicine and "alternative" and "complementary" medicine.

National Council Against Health Fraud

http://www.ncahf.org/
Non-profit voluntary health agency focusing on health fraud, misinformation, and quackery as public health concerns. Read their position papers on acupuncture, homepathy, chiropractic, and other health issues.

SURGERY

American College of Surgeons

http://www.facs.org/
Public information section offers guidelines on choosing a qualified surgeon.

Tests and Procedures - MedlinePlus

http://www.nlm.nih.gov/medlineplus/tutorial.html
Interactive tutorials on 24 common tests and diagnostic procedures and more than 30 surgeries and treatment procedures.

References

IMAGES

Arnold-Chiari Malformation

Basket of Puppies| Wikipedia.con

Photographs of the occipital bones:

"BodyParts3D, © The Database Center for Life Science licensed under CC Attribution-Share Alike 2.1 Japan."(Google translate)

CM and Syringomyelia: Holocord syringomyelia presenting as rapidly progressive foot drop

Saifudheen K, Jose J, Gafoor VA - J Neurosci Rural Pract (2011)

Ehlers-Danlos Syndrome Filipem|Wikipedia.com

Brainstem CFCF|Wikipedia.com

Occipital craniotomy scar. Ghasemi M, Golabchi K, Shaygannejad V, Rezvani M - J Res Med Sci (2011)

Other References

"Bobby Jones Society | Chiari & Syringomyelia Foundation". Csfinfo.org. Retrieved 2011-11-04.

"Boy's Brainstem Saved By A Nose". Columbia Medical Center Department of Neurological Surgery. Retrieved 2010-01-19.

"Chiari malformation". Dorlands Medical Dictionary.

"Chiari malformation: Symptoms". Mayo Clinic

"Cleveland Clinic Children's Hospital Pediatric Radiology Image Gallery". Cleveland Clinic. 2010. Archived from the original on 27 June 2010. Retrieved June 14, 2010.

"clinic_duty: House MD – 5.22 House Divided". Community.livejournal.com. Retrieved 2011-11-04.

"Code 453.0: Budd-Chiari Syndrome". 2008 ICD-9-CM Diagnosis.

"Congenital Chiari malformations". Neurology India 58 (1): 6–14. doi:10.4103/0028-3886.60387. PMID 20228456.

"Current Pain and Headache Reports, Volume 11, Number 1". SpringerLink. 2011-08-06. doi:10.1007/s11916-007-0022-x. Retrieved 2011-11-04.

"Department of Neurological Surgery - University of Washington". Depts.washington.edu. Retrieved 2011-11-04.

"Dr. Bland Discusses Chiari & EDS 4(10)". Conquerchiari.org. 2006-11-20. Retrieved 2011-11-04.

"Dysautonomia News - Winter/Spring 2006". Dinet.org. Retrieved 2011-11-04.

"Medscape: Medscape Access". Emedicine.medscape.com.

"Medscape: Medscape Access". Emedicine.medscape.com. Retrieved 2011-11-04.

"Neuroradiology - Chiari malformation (I-IV)".

"Rosanne Cash recovering from brain surgery - Entertainment - Celebrities - TODAY.com". MSNBC. 2011-10-26. Retrieved 2011-11-04.

Adams RD, Victor M: Principles of Neurology. New York, McGraw-Hill, Inc: 1100-1103, 1993

Adnan BURINA, Dževdet SMAJLOVIĆ, Osman SINANOVIĆ, Mirjana VIDOVIĆ, Omer Ć. IBRAHIMAGIĆ (2009). "ARNOLD–CHIARI MALFORMATION AND SYRINGOMYELIA". Acta Med Sal 38: 44–46.

Albers FW, Ingels KJ: Otoneurological manifestations in chiari 1 malformation. J Laryngol Otol 107: 441-443, 1993

Allen CD: Neurology of cervical spondylotic myelopathy, in Saundrs RL, Bernini PM (eds): Cervical Spondylotic Myelopathy. Boston, Blackwell Scientific Publications: 29-47, 1992

Atkinson JLD, Kokmen E, Miller GM: Evidence of posterior fossa hypoplasia in the familial variant of adult Chiari 1 malformation: Case report. Neurosurgery 42: 401-404, 1998

Ball PA, Saunders RL: Subjective Myelopathy, in Saunders RL, Bernini PM (eds): Cervical Spondylotic Myelopathy. Boston, Blackwell Scientific Publications: 48-55, 1992

Barnett GH, Hardy RW, Jr, Little JR, Bay JW, Sypert GW: Thoracic spinal canal stenosis. J Neurosurg 66: 338-344, 1987

Bondurant CP, Oro JJ: Spinal cord injury without radiographic abnormality and chiari malformation. J Neurosurg 79: 833-838, 1993

Bornstein D: Prevalence and treatment outcome of primary and secondary fibromyalgia in patients with spinal pain. Spine 20(7): 796-800, 1995

Brain WR, Northfield D, Wilkinson M: The neurological manifestations of cervical spondylosis. Brain 75: 187-225, 1952

Cammalleri R, D'Amelio M, Gangitano M, Raimondo D, Rossetti M, Camarda R: Monosymptomatic presentation of type 1 Arnold-Chiari malformation: report of two cases. Ital J Neurol Sci 15: 57-60, 1994

Chiari Malformation Fact Sheet. National Institute of Neurological Disorders and Stroke Web site. 2009;http://www.ninds.nih.gov/disorders/chiari/detail_chiari.htm.

Chiari Malformation Fact Sheet. NINDS. February 1, 2012;http://www.ninds.nih.gov/disorders/chiari/detail_chiari.htm#194173087

Clarke E, Robinson PK: Cervical myelopathy: a complication of cervical spondylosis. Brain 79: 483-510, 1956

Clauw, DJ: Fibromyalgia: more than just a musculoskeletal disease. Am Fam Physician 52(3):843-51, 853-4, 1995

Clinical evidence for cervical myelopathy due to Chiari malformation and spinal stenosis in a non-randomized group of patients with the diagnosis of fibromyalgia

CNN. Don't get hurt by an MRI. http://thechart.blogs.cnn.com/2011/10/26/dont-get-hurt-by-an-mri/comment-page-3/

Dan S. Heffez, Ruth E. Ross, [...], and Charity G. Moore

de Barros MC, Farias W, Ataide L, Lins S: Basilar impression and Arnold-Chiari malformation. J Neuro Neurosurg Psychiat 31: 596-605, 1968

de Jesus M: Fibromyalgia onset. Am J Nurs 100(1): 14, 2000

Denno JJ, Meadows GR: Early diagnosis of cervical spondylotic myelopathy. A useful clinical sign. Spine 16: 1353-1355, 1991

Donald F, Esdaile JM, Kimoff JR, Fitzcharles MA: Muscloskeletal complaints and fibromyalgia in patients attending a respiratory sleep disorders clinic. J Rheumatol 23(9): 1612-6, 1996

Dyste GN, Menezes AH, Van Gilder JC: Symptomatic Chiari malformations: An analysis of presentation, management, and long-term outcome. J Neurosurg 71: 159-168, 1989

Fender FA: A new hazard of cervical laminectomy. JAMA 149: 227-228, 1952

Girard PF, Garde A, Devic M: Contribution a l'etude anatomique des manifestation medullaires observees au cours des discarthroses. Rev Neurol 90: 481954

Guo F, Wang M, Long J, et al. (2007). "Surgical management of Chiari malformation: analysis of 128 cases". Pediatr Neurosurg 43 (5): 375–81.doi:10.1159/000106386. PMID 17786002.

Homes G: Pain of Central Origin: Contributions to medical and biological research dedicated to Si William Osler. New York, Paul B. Hoeber, Inc: 235-246, 1919

J. Klekamp, U. Batzdorf, M. Samii and H. W. Bothe (1996). "The surgical treatment of Chiari I malformation". Acta Neurochirurgica 138 (7): 788–801. doi:10.1007/BF01411256. PMID 8869706.

James DS: Significance of chronic tonsillar herniation in sudden death. Forensic Sci Int 75: 217-223, 1995

Jason LA, Taylor RR, Kennedy CL: Chronic fatigue syndrome, fibromyalgia, and multiple chemical sensitivities in a community-based sample of persons with chronic fatigue syndrome-like symptoms. Psychosom Med 62(5): 655-63, 2000

Johnson GD, Harbaugh RE, Lenz SB: Surgical decompression of chiari 1 malformation for isolated progressive sensorineural hearing loss. Am J Otol 15: 634-638, 1994

Johnston I, Hawke S, Halmagyi M, Teo C. The pseudotumor syndrome. Disorders of cerebrospinal fluid circulation causing intracranial hypertension without ventriculomegaly. Arch Neurol 1991;48:740-747.

Kaipo T. Pau. "Chapter XVIII.16. Developmental Brain Anomalies". In Jeffrey K. Okamoto et al. Case Based Pediatrics For Medical Students and Residents.

Kaplan L, Kennedy F: Effect of head position on manometrics of cerebrospinal fluid in cervical lesions: a new diagnostic test. Brain 73: 337-345, 1950

Kojima A, Mayanagi K, Okui S (February 2009). "Progression of pre-existing Chiari type I malformation secondary to cerebellar hemorrhage: case report". Neurol. Med. Chir. (Tokyo) 49 (2): 90–2. doi:10.2176/nmc.49.90.PMID 19246872.[dead link]

Korszun A: Sleep and circadian rhythm disorders in fibromyalgia. Curr Rheumatol Rep 2(2): 124-30, 2000

Kremer M: Sitting, standing and walking: part 2. Brit MJ 2: 1211958

Kulisevsky J, Avila A, Grau-Veciana JM: Isolated lingual myoclonus associated with an Arnold-Chiari malformation [letter]. J Neurol Neurosurg Psychiatry 57: 660-661, 1994

Kurland JE, Coyle WJ, Winkler A, Zable E: Prevalence of irritable bowel syndrome and depression in fibromyalgia. Dig Dis Sci 51(3):454-60, 2006

Ladd AL, Scranton PE: Congenital cervical stenosis presenting as transient quadriplegia in athletes. Report of two cases. J Bone Joint Surg [AM] 68: 1371-1374, 1986

l-Allaf AW, Dunbar KL, Hallum NS, Nosratzadeh B, Templeton KD, Pullar T: A case-control study examining the role of physical trauma in the onset of fibromyalgia syndrome. Rheumatology 41(4): 450-3, 2002

Langfitt TW, Elliot FA: Pain in the back and legs caused by cervical spinal cord compression. JAMA 200: 382-385, 1967

Langfitt TW: Cervical spondylosis: the neurological mimic. WV Med J 65: 97-100, 1969

Li-Gang Cui, Ling Jiang, Hua-Bin Zhang, Bin Liu, Jin-Rui Wang, Jian-Wen Jiaa, Wen Chen (2011). "Monitoring of cerebrospinal fluid flow by intraoperative ultrasound in patients with Chiari I malformation". Clinical Neurology and Neurosurgery 113 (3): 173–176.doi:10.1016/j.clineuro.2010.10.011. PMID 21075511.

Loft LM, Ward RF: Hiccups: A case presentation an etiologic review. Arch Otolaryngol Head Neck Surg 118: 1115-1119, 1992

Loukas M, Shayota BJ, Oelhafen K, Miller JH, Chern JJ, Tubbs RS, Oakes WJ (2011). "Associated disorders of Chiari Type I malformations: a review".Neurosurg Focus 31 (3): E3. doi:10.3171/2011.6.FOCUS11112.PMID 21882908.

Lowman RM, Finkelstein A: Air myelography for demonstration of the cervical spinal cord. Radiology 39: 700-706, 1942

Lundsford LD, Bissonette D, Zorub D: Anterior surgery for cervical disc disease. Part 2. J Neurosurg 53: 12-19, 1980

Marcus DA, Bernstein C, Rudy TE: Fibromyalgia and headache: an epidemiological study supporting migraine as part of the fibromyalgia syndrome. Clin Rheumatol 24(6): 595-601, 2005

Massimo Caldarelli, Concezio Di Rocco (2004). "Diagnosis of Chiari I malformation and related syringomyelia: radiological and neurophysiological studies". Childs Nerv Syst 20 (5): 332–335. doi:10.1007/s00381-003-0880-4. PMID 15034729.

Matsumoto T, Symon L: Surgicial management of syringomyelia- Current results. Surg Neurol 32: 258-265, 1989

Matsumoto Y: Concept and therapy for fibromyalgia. Nippon Naika Gakkai Zasshi 95(3): 510-5, 2006

Matsunaga S, Sakou T, Imamura T, Morimoto N: Dissociated motor loss in the upper extremities. Clinical features and pathophysiology. Spine 18: 1964-1967, 1993

Matsuoka A, Shitara T, Okamoto M, Sano H: Transient deafness with iopamidol following angiography. Acta Otolaryngol Suppl 541: 78-80, 1994

McComas CF, Frost JL, Schochet SS: Posttraumatic syringomyelia with paroxysmal episodes of unconsciousness. Arch Neurol 40: 322-324, 1983

Mehalic TF, Pezzuli RT, Applebaum BI: Magnetic resonance imaging and cervical spondylotic myelopathy. Neurosurgery 26: 217-227, 1990

Middleton GS, Teacher JH: Injury of the spinal cord due to rupture of an intervertebral disc during muscular effort. Glasglow Med J 76: 1-6, 1911

Milhorat TH, Bolognese PA, Nishikawa M, McDonnell NB, Francomano CA (December 2007). "Syndrome of occipitoatlantoaxial hypermobility, cranial settling, and chiari malformation type I in patients with hereditary disorders of connective tissue". Journal of Neurosurgery: Spine 7 (6): 601–9. doi:10.3171/SPI-07/12/601. PMID 18074684.

Milhorat TH, Capacelli AL, Jr, Anzil AP, Kotzen RM, Milhorat RM: Pathological basis of spinal cord cavitation in syringomyelia: analysis of 105 autopsy cases. J Neurosurg 82: 802-812, 1994

Morgan D, Williams B: syringobulbia a surgical appraisal. J Neuro Neurosurg Psychiat 55: 1132-1141, 1992

MRI Dainali | Wikimedia Commons

Mueller DM and Oro JJ, J. Am. Acad. Nurs. Pract., Vol. 16, Issue 2, pp 134-8, March 2004.

Neumann L, Buskila, D: Epidemiology of fibromyalgia. Curr Pain Headache Rep 7(5): 362-8, 2003

Neurological References

Nohria V, Oakes WJ: Chiari 1 malformation: A review of 43 patients. Pediatr Neurosurg 16: 222-227, 1990

O'Connell JEA: Involvement of spinal cord by intervertebral disc protrusions. Brit J Surg 43: 225-247, 1955

O'Shaughnessy BA, Bendok BR, Parkinson RJ, et al. (January 2006)."Acquired Chiari malformation Type I associated with a supratentorial arteriovenous malformation. Case report and review of the literature". J. Neurosurg. 104 (1 Suppl): 28–32. doi:10.3171/ped.2006.104.1.28.PMID 16509477.

Parker HL, Adson AW: Compression of the spinal cord and its roots by hypertrophic osteo-arthritis. Surg Gynecol Obstet 41: 1-14, 1925

Peres MF, Young WB, Kaup AO, Zukerman E, Silberstein SD: Fibromyalgia is common in patients with transformed migraine. Neurology 57(7;):1326-8, 2001

Petersen MC, Wolraich M, Sherbondy A, Wagener J: Abnormalities in control of ventilation in newborn infants with myelomeningocele. J Pediatr 126: 1011-1015, 1995

Peyman Pakzaban. Chiari Malformation. eMedicine. March 2, 2012;http://emedicine.medscape.com/article/1483583-overview.

Pidcock FS, Sandel ME, Faro S: Late onset syringomyelia after traumatic brain injury: association with chiari 1 malformation. Arch Phys Med Rehabil 75: 695-698, 1994

Pillay PK, Awad IA, Little JR, Hahn JF: Symptomatic Chiari malformation in adults: A new classification based on magnetic resonance imaging with clinical and prognostic significance. Neurosurgery 28: 639-645, 1991

Pujol J, Roig, C, Capdevila A, Pou A, Marti-Vilalta JL, Kulisevsky J, Escartin A, Zannoli G: Motion of the cerebellar tonsils in chiari type 1 malformation studied by cine phase-contrast MRI. Neurology 45: 1746-1753, 1995

Raftopoulos C, Sanchez A, Matos C, Baleriaux D, Bank WO, Brotchi J: Hydrosyringomyelia-Chiari 1 complex. Prospective evaluation of a modified foramen magnum decompression procedure: Preliminary results. Surg Neurol 39: 163-169, 1992

Rhodus NL, Fricton J, Carlson P, Messner R: Oral symptoms associated with fibromyalgia syndrome. J Rheumatol 30(8): 1841-5, 2003

Rosenbaum, RB; DP Ciaverella (2004). Neurology in Clinical Practice. Butterworth Heinemann. pp. 2192–2193. ISBN 0-7506-7469-5.

Rutkove SB, Matheson JK, Logigian EL: Restless legs syndrome in patients with polyneuropathy. Muscle Nerve 19(5): 670-2, 1996

Saez RJ, Onofrio BM, Yanagihara T: Experience with Arnold-Chiari malformation, 1960 to 1970. J Neurosurg 45: 416-422, 1976

Schneider RC, Cherry GR, Pantek H: Syndrome of acute central cervical spinal cord injury with special reference to mechanisms involved in hypertension injuries of cervical spine. J Neurosurg 11: 546-577, 1954

Shaver JL, Wilbur J, Robinson FP, Wang E, Buntin MS: Womens health issues with fibromyalgia syndrome. J Womens Health 15(9):1035-45, 2006

Simmons Z, Biller J, Beck DW, Keyes W: Painless compressive cervical myelopathy with false localizing sensory findings. Spine 11: 869-872, 1986

Stahl SM: Fibromyalgia: the enigma and the stigma. J Clin Psychiatry 62(7): 501-2, 2001

Sudou K, Tashiro K: Segmental hyperhidrosis in syringomyelia with chiari malformation. J Neurol 240: 75-78, 1993

Symonds C: Interrelation of trauma and cervical spondylosis in compression of cercival cord. Lancet 1: 451-454, 1953

Tatlow WFT, Bammer HC: Syndrome of vertebral artery compression. Neurology 7: 331-340, 1957

Tikiz C, Muezzinoglu T, Pirildar T, Taskn EO, Frat A, Tuzun C: Sexual dysfunction in female subjects with fibromyalgia. J Urol 174(2):620-3, 2005

Todd C. Hankinson, Eli Grunstein, Paul Gardner, Theodore J. Spinks, and Richard C. E. Anderson (2010). "Transnasal odontoid resection followed by posterior decompression and occipitocervical fusion in children with Chiari malformation Type I and ventral brainstem compression". J Neurosurg Pediatrics 5 (6): 549–553. doi:10.3171/2010.2.PEDS09362.

Torg JS: Cervical spinal stenosis with cord neurapraxia and transient quadriplegia. Clin Sports Med 9: 279-296, 1990

van Alphen HAM: Migraine, a result of increased CSF pressure: a new pathophysiological concept (preliminary report). Neurosurg Rev 9: 121-124, 1986

Van den Bergh R, Van Calenbergh F: Headache and headache-attacks in the chiari 1 malformation and in syringomyelia. Headache Quarterly 8: 15-21, 1997

Vannemreddy P, Nourbakhsh A, Willis B, Guthikonda B. (January 2010).

Visuri T, Lindhom H, Lindqvist A, Dahlstrom S, Viljanen A: Cardiovascular functional disorder in primary fibromyalgia: a noninvasive study in 17 young men. Arthritis Care Res 5(4): 210-5, 1992

Weir PT, Harlan GA, Nkoy FL, Jones SS, Hegmann KT, Gren LH, Lyon JL: The incidence of fibromyalgia and its associated comorbidities: a population-based retrospective cohort study based on International Classification of Diseases, 9th Revision codes. J Clin Rheumatol 12(3): 124-8, 2006

Weissbecker I, Floyd A, Dedert E, Salmon P, Sephton S: Childhood trauma and diurnal cortisol disruption in fibromyalgia syndrome. Psychoneuroendocrinology 31(3): 312-24, 2006

White KP, Harth M: Classification, epidemiology, and natural history of fibromyalgia. Curr Pain Headache Rep 5(4): 320-9, 2001

Wolfe F, Ross K, Anderson J, Russell IJ: Aspects of fibromyalgia in the general population: sex, pain threshold, and fibromyalgia symptoms. J Rheuomatol 22(1): 151-6, 1995

Yap KB, Lieu PK, Chia HP, Menon EB, Tan ES: Outcome of patients with cervical spondylotic myelopathy seen at a rehabilitation centre. Singapore Med J 34: 237-240, 1993

Yu YL, Woo E, Huang CY: Cervical spondylotic myelopathy and radiculopathy. Acta Neurol Scand 75: 367-373, 1987

Yunus MB, Aldag JC: Restless legs syndrome and leg cramps in fibromyalgia syndrome: a controlled study. BMJ 312:1339, 1996

Yunus MB: Gender differences in fibromyalgia and other related syndromes. J Gend Specif Med 5(2): 42-7, 2002

CPSIA information can be obtained
at www.ICGtesting.com
Printed in the USA
FSOW04n0750080517
34005FS